Fourth Edition

UNIPAC 3

Assessing and Treating Pain

Sharon M. Weinstein, MD FAAHPM
Huntsman Cancer Institute at the
    University of Utah
Salt Lake City, UT

Russell K. Portenoy, MD
Beth Israel Medical Center
MJHS Hospice and Palliative Care
New York, NY

Sarah E. Harrington, MD
University of Arkansas for Medical Sciences
Little Rock, AR

Reviewed by
Paul Sloan, MD
University of Kentucky College of Medicine
Lexington, KY

Edited by
C. Porter Storey, Jr., MD FACP FAAHPM
Colorado Permanente Medical Group
Executive Vice President
American Academy of Hospice and Palliative
    Medicine
Boulder, CO

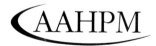

American Academy of Hospice and Palliative Medicine
4700 W. Lake Avenue
Glenview, IL 60025-1485
aahpm.org | PalliativeDoctors.org

The information presented and opinions expressed herein are those of the editor and authors and do not necessarily represent the views of the American Academy of Hospice and Palliative Medicine. Any recommendations made by the editor and authors must be weighed against the healthcare provider's own clinical judgment, based on but not limited to such factors as the patient's condition, benefits versus risks of suggested treatment, and comparison with recommendations of pharmaceutical compendia and other medical and palliative care authorities. Published in the United States by the American Academy of Hospice and Palliative Medicine, 4700 W. Lake Avenue, Glenview, IL 60025-1485.

Publishing Staff
Julie Bruno, Senior Education Manager
Angie Forbes, Education Manager
Jerrod Liveoak, Senior Managing Editor
Katie Macaluso, Managing Editor
Monica Piotrowski, Assistant Editor
Sonya Jones, Senior Designer
Stephanie Euzebio, Graphic Designer
Cover design and page layout by Stephanie Euzebio

ISBN 978-1-889296-43-2

Contents

Tables

Figures

Acknowledgments

The editor, authors, contributors, and the American Academy of Hospice and Palliative Medicine are deeply grateful to all who have participated in the development of this component of the *UNIPAC: A Resource for Hospice and Palliative Care Professionals* self-study program. The expertise of the contributors and reviewers involved in the previous and current editions of the *UNIPACs* has greatly improved their value and contents. Our special thanks are extended to the original authors of this book, C. Porter Storey, Jr., MD FACP FAAHPM, and Carol F. Knight, EdM; the pharmacist reviewer for *UNIPAC 3*, James B. Ray, PharmD; the reviewer for the *UNIPAC 3 amplifire* confidence-based learning module, Holly Yang, MD FAAHPM; the authors of the previous edition of *UNIPAC 3*, Andrea Bial, MD, and Stacie Levine, MD; and the many professionals who volunteered their time and expertise to review the content and test this program in the field—Timothy E. Quill, MD FACP FAAHPM; Katherine Juba, PharmD BCPS; Joseph W. Shega, MD; Judith A. Paice, PhD RN; Linda King, MD; Perry Fine, MD; John W. Finn, MD FAAHPM; Gerald H. Holman, MD FAAFP; Eli N. Perencevich, DO; and Julia L. Smith, MD.

Continuing Medical Education

Purpose

A *UNIPAC* is a packet of information formatted as an independent-study program. It includes practical clinical scenarios to orient the reader to the material, educational content, and references. This independent-study program is intended for healthcare providers who are interested in incorporating the principles of hospice and palliative medicine into their daily practice. It is designed to increase competence in palliative care interventions for improving a patient's quality of life. Specific, practical information is presented to help physicians and other practitioners assess and manage selected problems. After reading the *UNIPAC*, practitioners are encouraged to complete a separate online confidence-based learning module. Physicians may only obtain *AMA PRA Category 1 Credits*™ by completing this module.

Learning Objectives

Upon completion of this continuing medical education (CME) program, a physician should be better able to

- assess for the presence of cancer-related and noncancer-related (nonmalignant) pain
- identify physical, emotional, social, and spiritual aspects of pain and suffering
- differentiate nociceptive and neuropathic pain
- calculate an appropriate starting dose of morphine for opioid-naive patients
- make safe and effective conversions from one opioid to another and from one route of drug administration to another
- prescribe appropriate treatments for common side effects such as nausea and constipation associated with opioid use
- prescribe appropriate nonopioid adjuvant drugs to treat nociceptive and neuropathic pain
- manage acute and procedural pain
- be familiar with nonpharmacologic pain management strategies
- be familiar with the needs of special populations.

Disclosure

In accordance with the Accreditation Council for Continuing Medical Education's Standards for Commercial Support, all CME providers are required to disclose to the activity audience the relevant financial relationships of the planners, reviewers, and authors involved in the development of CME content. An individual has a relevant financial relationship if he or she has a financial relationship in any amount occurring in the last 12 months with a commercial interest whose products or services are discussed in the CME activity content over which the individual has control. AAHPM requires that all relevant financial relationships be resolved prior to planning or participating in the activity. **The authors, editor, and reviewers for this module have disclosed no relevant financial relationships, with the following exceptions.**

Sharon M. Weinstein, MD FAAHPM, was on the advisory board for Archimedes Pharmaceuticals and received compensation for a speaking engagement for Optum Health. **Russell K. Portenoy, MD,** disclosed financial relationships with Cephalon, CNSBio, Covidien Mallinckrodt Inc, Grupo Ferrer, Purdue Pharma, and Xenon; he has received educational/research grants from Ameritox, Archimedes Pharmaceuticals, Cephalon, Covidien Mallinckrodt Inc, Endo Pharmaceuticals, Forest Labs, GW Pharma, King Pharma, Meda Pharmaceuticals, Ortho-McNeil Janssen Scientific Affairs LLD, Otsuka Pharma, Purdue Pharma, and the Tempur-Pedic Corporation.

Term of Offering

The release date for the *UNIPAC 3 **amplifire*** module is April 1, 2012, and the expiration date is March 31, 2015.

Introduction

Patients with serious or life-threatening illnesses have varied primary diseases and comorbidities, diverse illness trajectories, and a rapidly changing therapeutic landscape. The burden of serious illness is high for both patients and families, and symptom distress contributes substantially to this burden. Chronic pain is among the most important of symptoms in terms of prevalence and potential impact, and integrating pain management best practices into humane, effective, and affordable palliative care is a key challenge for healthcare systems worldwide.

Although much progress has been achieved in our ability to control pain, many patients continue to endure unrelieved pain, especially during the last months of life. At the end of life, 62% to 90% of children report pain.[1] Of patients with noncancer diagnoses (eg, congestive heart failure, cirrhosis), more than 40% experience severe pain within days of death.[2] A 2007 systematic review found a 64% prevalence of pain in metastatic or advanced stage cancer, and a rating of moderate or severe pain intensity in more than one-third of these patients.[3] In all populations with solid tumors the overall prevalence of clinically significant chronic pain ranges from 15% to more than 75%, depending on the type and extent of disease and many other factors.[4]

Numerous treatment guidelines have been published during the past quarter century,[5-13] and limited data and extensive clinical experience suggest adherence to these guidelines yields satisfactory relief for most patients.[14] Unfortunately, multiple barriers to effective treatments result in outcomes that are not always optimal.[15] Indeed, a 2008 review suggested that an average of 43% of patients with cancer receive inappropriate care for pain.[16,17] These data affirm the continuing need for professional education in pain management.

Pain is often a component of suffering during serious illness. *Suffering* can be defined as "the state of severe distress associated with events that threaten the intactness of the person."[18] Suffering occurs when patients perceive the impending destruction of their personhood, and it continues until the threat of disintegration has passed or until the patient's integrity can be restored.[19] Suffering in the context of serious illness has been termed *total pain*, a concept based on the recognition of pain as an integrated biopsychosocial and existential construct (**Table 1**). The four components of total pain are
- physical pain
- emotional or psychic pain
- social or interpersonal pain
- spiritual or existential pain.

Wilson and colleagues found that more than 25% of patients with advanced illness rated their suffering as moderate to severe, and although physical pain was most commonly associated with the experience of suffering, all four components of total pain were significant.[20] Emotional, spiritual, and social pain may be caused by conditions such as anxiety, depression, isolation and loneliness, and fear. Family concerns add to a patient's burden. Terminally ill patients may also

---

Table 1. Elements in the Domains of Total Pain

P   **Physical** problems, often multiple, must be specifically diagnosed and treated.

A   **Anxiety**, anger, and depression are critical components of pain that must be addressed by the physician, in cooperation with other healthcare professionals.

I   **Interpersonal** problems including loneliness, financial stress, and family tensions are often interwoven into the fabric of a patient's symptoms.

N   **Not accepting** approaching death, a sense of hopelessness, and a desperate search for meaning can cause severe suffering that is unrelieved by medications.

experience financial concerns, a loss of faith, and loss of meaning.

Although a model of total pain that links distress in the physical, social, emotional, and spiritual domains emphasizes the multifaceted nature of pain, it may unintentionally reinforce the erroneous view that pain is either physical or nonphysical. This view reflects a reductionist medical model that can distract from a more holistic perspective that better reflects the core precepts of palliative care. It is important to acknowledge that pain from an obvious physical source always has a psychological component, and likewise, a multidimensional pain experience in a patient with serious illness often is related to numerous other factors that may contribute to the broader construct of suffering. Based on clinical experience, it appears likely that pain that is explainable, is expected to be transitory, and has meaning (such as pain associated with medical procedures) contributes less to suffering than pain that is persistent, has an unknown source, and occurs without meaning. Pain and suffering both require careful assessment (see *UNIPAC 2*).

Efforts to relieve pain are usually welcomed, but clinical interventions may not adequately improve quality of life or reduce suffering if they are pursued separately from the "whole person" concerns associated with a serious or life-threatening illness. This therapeutic framework is sometimes termed *supportive care*, particularly in oncology settings, but more generally it is understood as the foundation for palliative care. Generalist palliative care, including a focus on pain management, should be a best practice for all clinicians contributing to the care of patients. Specialist palliative care provided by an interdisciplinary team should be available when problems, which may include pain, are complex and severe.[21]

Although analgesic drug therapy is usually a priority in patients with moderate or severe pain that is complicating serious or life-threatening illness, there is always value in considering a multimodality approach that may incorporate disease-modifying treatments that target the etiology of pain and a variety of nonpharmacologic interventions for pain or other sources of suffering. Opioid-based pharmacotherapy is, however, the main strategy for pain treatment in populations with active life-threatening disease. Surveys indicate that opioid-based pharmacotherapy can provide adequate relief to as many as 90% of those with cancer pain,[22,23] and the guidelines developed for cancer pain have been applied to pain associated with numerous other serious conditions such as HIV/AIDS and sickle cell disease.

Given the potential for a high rate of success, the finding that unrelieved pain remains common in medically ill populations can be attributed, in part, to undertreatment. A study of pain associated with HIV disease is illustrative: Hospitalized patients with pain were receiving daily physician visits, but their pain remained uncontrolled; after consultation by a specialist pain team, oral morphine was ordered on a 24-hour schedule and the results were described as dramatically favorable.[24]

Why would a specialist team be needed to initiate a simple and common analgesic technique? Pain may be undertreated for several reasons. Patients' and families' concerns about opioid analgesics, lack of professional education and persistent misconceptions about the risks of opioid therapy, and professionals' fear of regulatory scrutiny all may contribute. Analgesic drug availability also may pose a significant problem. Those who are providing specialist palliative care to patients with chronic pain must be aware of these barriers and work to remove them, both in managing individual cases and in the broader context of health care.[25]

Effective pain management may be conceptualized as a continuous multistep process: (1)

thorough assessment of all types of pain a patient is experiencing and evaluation of potential benefits versus risks of various treatment modalities; (2) treatment of each type of pain with an individualized plan of care that may include both etiology-specific and symptomatic interventions; and (3) continuous reassessment of treatment goals (eg, pain level, functional goals, sleep, mood, social interaction, etc.) and evaluation of the overall balance between treatment benefit and adverse effects. When pain increases or remains uncontrolled, a thorough reassessment should be performed and, based on these findings, a prompt plan readjustment should be made.

There is an important and emerging consensus that the approach to pain in many populations with serious or life-threatening illness is fundamentally different than the conventional approach to chronic nonmalignant pain syndromes. The modifier *nonmalignant* has been used in the clinical literature to describe pain not associated with life-threatening conditions such as cancer. Palliative care clinicians must understand that this label does not imply the pain experience is well tolerated or unassociated with potentially severe consequences, and some patients with pain syndromes typically subsumed under this label should be treated as though they have a progressive incurable disorder that warrants a palliative care approach. When this descriptor is used in discussions of policy or guideline development, however, it usually refers to highly prevalent conditions commonly encountered in primary care and not associated with reduced survival.

More than 100 million Americans experience chronic pain.[26] Headache and lower back pain are the most common types of pain in developed countries. Nine of 10 Americans experience at least one headache annually, and more than 25 million Americans have recurrent migraines. Two-thirds of Americans have back pain during their lifetimes, and more than 26 million between the ages of 20 and 64 years experience frequent back pain. Other common conditions include arthritis, neuropathic pain syndromes such as diabetic neuropathy, and fibromyalgia. Chronic painful conditions in the developing world are more likely to be related to malnutrition, infectious diseases, and trauma, including limb amputation, which affect millions of the world's inhabitants.

Palliative care providers are strong advocates for quality of life and may be called upon to contribute to the care of patients with varied types of chronic nonmalignant pain (**Table 2**). Accordingly, palliative care providers should have a general understanding of the approach to common types of chronic nonmalignant pain.

Table 2. Decision Analysis: Chronic Nonmalignant Pain[27]

1. Recognize that the conventional therapeutic approach to most chronic nonmalignant pain will not mirror the preferred strategy to address pain in patients with advanced illness.
2. If contributing to the care of patients with chronic nonmalignant pain, become familiar with the disorder in question and understand the options for etiology-based and multimodality symptomatic therapy.
3. When patients have chronic nonmalignant pain, recognize that long-term opioid therapy is the mainstay approach only when patients have active serious illness and in other situations is considered case by case and usually only after other therapies prove ineffective.
4. Identify the clinician who will be primarily responsible for the care of a patient, including the care of his or her pain, and clarify roles and responsibilities of palliative care team members and other providers, particularly regarding the prescribing of controlled prescription drugs.

Adapted from Nonmalignant Pain in Palliative Medicine (p. 931), by S Weinstein, in D Walsh, R Fainsinger, K Foley, et al. (Eds.), Palliative Medicine, 2009, Philadelphia: Saunders. © 2009 by Elsevier. Reprinted with permission.

Pain Pathophysiology and Nomenclature

The ability to perceive and react to noxious stimuli is a necessary function of the nervous system. Acute pain occurs when the nervous system is functioning normally to transmit information about injurious events in the environment or in the body. Pain is pathological when it is no longer signaling noxious events or when it becomes associated with damaging physical or psychological outcomes. When pain persists beyond several months, it usually is pathological, regardless of whether there are persistent noxious stimuli. When pain becomes chronic, it is best considered to be an illness in its own right.

The International Association for the Study of Pain defines *pain* as "an unpleasant sensory and emotional experience associated with actual or potential tissue damage, or described in terms of such damage."[28] In the normal course of events, pain occurs in association with potentially damaging stimuli, which are detected by peripheral nociceptors (A-delta and C-fibers) located in skin, muscle, joint, and visceral tissues. Nociceptors have varied receptors and channels that may respond to different types of noxious stimuli; some of these neurons are polymodal, some are modality specific, and some are "silent" until specific conditions (such as local inflammation) occur. Nociceptors transduce stimuli into electrical signals that are transmitted to the dorsal horn of the spinal cord, where complex neurophysiological and neurochemical processes occur. These processes are mediated by segmental neurons and descending pathways from higher centers. Signals that enter the dorsal horn may or may not be transmitted through ascending neural pathways to the thalamus, limbic areas, and areas of the cerebral cortex.

The multiple endogenous mechanisms that process and modulate incoming nociceptive signals are exceedingly complex. They presumably are the neurophysiologic underpinning to the reality that human pain has both sensory discriminative dimensions and affective and cognitive dimensions.

The endorphin system is among the important endogenous systems modulating the perception of pain. Endorphins, which comprise many compounds (such as the enkephalins, dynorphin, and beta endorphin), are the endogenous ligands for a complex array of opioid receptors. There are three major classes of opioid receptors—mu, kappa, and delta. These receptors are located in many nonneural tissues and in both the peripheral nervous system and central nervous system (CNS). Receptors involved in pain modulation inhibit calcium flux and affect the release of neurotransmitters that determine the balance between pronociceptive and antinociceptive neurotransmission.

Pathophysiology of Chronic Pain

When pain becomes chronic there are changes in the physiologic systems for transduction of information about noxious events, transmission of information proximally, and modulation of this information at multiple levels. Advances in neuroscience research that have begun to elucidate pain-related genomics and the many aspects of neuroplasticity provide a glimpse into the extraordinary complexity of the many mechanisms that may contribute to human pain. Animal studies have shown that afferent input from noxious events can lead to physiological and morphological changes such as remodeling of neural arborization, creating new circuits or strengthening old ones, forming new active zones along existing axons, and changing the structure of dendrites to improve the propagation of postsynaptic potentials to integrative zones. Both membrane excitability and synaptic transmission are enhanced in sensory neurons with damaged axons. Signal proteins synthesized in response to such sensitization are probably distributed throughout the neuronal arbor and consequently affect structural remodeling. Perception is encoded in both anatomical structures and temporal patterns of neural activity in the brain, and studies of long-term potentiation exemplify the ways in which neural activity itself causes changes in synaptic connectivity.

Some chronic pain may be primarily attributable to prolonged tissue injury, accompanying inflammatory processes in the periphery, and peripheral sensitization of afferent neurons, and some may be primarily the result of sensitization of central neurons. Pain is a dynamic state and the mechanisms may evolve over time. Structural and functional changes of peripheral and central neurons occur with repeated noxious stimuli, persistent damaging stimuli, or direct injury to the nervous system itself. Glial-derived signaling molecules also can contribute to and modulate pain signaling in the spinal cord, and chronic pain in humans may be attributable to pathological functioning of a damaged nervous system at any level.[29]

The complex pathophysiology of clinical pain means that ongoing tissue damage need not be present for a patient to experience pain. When pain appears to be excessive for the degree of identifiable tissue damage, occult nociceptive processes or neuropathic mechanisms may be sustaining it, or processes that are primarily psychological are amplifying the pain. Although psychological processes profoundly influence pain expression and function, the term *psychogenic pain*, which refers to a syndrome that is primarily attributed to psychological factors and is identified as a psychiatric disorder, is rarely encountered in palliative care settings. Most patients with serious illnesses develop chronic pain as the result of obvious etiologies associated with damage to somatic, visceral, or neural structures, usually with multiple pathophysiologic mechanisms occurring simultaneously.

Pain Assessment

An effort to identify and characterize the etiology of the pain is a key element of a pain assessment. The etiology is a verifiable lesion or disorder that is likely to be perpetuating pain through direct tissue injury or a related process such as inflammation. Once identified, the etiology may suggest disease-modifying therapy for analgesic purposes, such as radiation to a bony metastasis, or it may redefine the extent of disease.

A pain assessment should also attempt to characterize pain according to clinically accepted inferences about the broad types of mechanisms sustaining the pain. In the setting of serious illness, the latter mechanisms usually are classified as "nociceptive," "neuropathic," or mixed. Although basic research in bone pain[30] and pain as the result of nerve injury[31] indicate that pathophysiologic labels applied in clinical settings oversimplify complex mechanisms, this classification, combined with syndrome identification, can be useful in practice.[32]

Nociceptive Pain

Nociceptive pain may be somatic or visceral and is associated with actual or potential tissue damage, which is believed to cause ongoing activation of intact nociceptors.[33] Inflammatory pain, a subtype, is sometimes distinguished on the basis of identifiable inflammation that presumably results in nociceptor activation.

Maggie

Maggie is a 65-year-old female with a history of metastatic breast cancer. She had a right total mastectomy with lymph node dissection and now has a single metastasis to her fourth lumbar vertebrae. She is undergoing cisplatin-based chemotherapy and radiation and is referred to a palliative care clinic for help with pain management. Maggie is tearful and shares multiple complaints that include constant dull aching pain in her lower back, chest wall pain at the site of her mastectomy, and sharp shooting pain down her right arm. She describes numbness and tingling in both hands and feet since starting the chemotherapy and has new onset right arm lymphedema. She tearfully reports that her pain has negatively affected her mood, sleep, and appetite. Maggie is fearful that her disease is progressing because her pain has not improved. The resident who is rotating with you asks, "Where do we start with this patient?"

When approaching a patient with multiple sources of pain the following questions may be helpful:

- Does she have acute or chronic pain (or a combination of the two)?
- Based on her history, what are the likely physiological etiologies of her pain?

- How would you characterize her pain? Does she have somatic, visceral, or neuropathic components?
- Does she have identifiable pain syndromes from either the cancer or cancer-related treatments (chemotherapy, radiation, surgery)?

The Case Continues

Maggie shares with you that her husband left her after hearing her diagnosis, and she is experiencing a great deal of frustration and loneliness. Her children live out of state, and she doesn't want to "bother" her friends. She becomes tearful in the office and says, "I just don't understand why this is happening to me. What did I do to deserve this misery?"

- Are there elements of her history that point to the following types of pain?
  - Emotional pain
  - Social pain
  - Spiritual pain
- How can you explore areas of total pain in Maggie's case?
- How difficult is it to explore these other areas if Maggie's physical pain is untreated or undertreated?

Somatic Pain

Somatic pain is caused by injury to the skin, other soft tissues, bones, or joints. Deep somatic pain is typically localized and described as aching, stabbing, throbbing, or "squeezing." Superficial somatic pain is usually sharper and may have a burning or pricking sensation. Examples of somatic pain include arthritis, wounds, and tumor invasion of soft tissues. Metastatic bone disease typically is labeled as somatic nociceptive pain, notwithstanding the emerging data

demonstrating a fundamental neuropathic process involved in at least some types.[30] Bone pain intensifies with movement (especially weight bearing), is often tender to palpation, and is often described as deep and aching. Bone pain requires a particularly careful assessment.[34] If there is severe pain during any weight-bearing activity, a radiograph may reveal an actual or potential pathologic fracture for which orthopedic stabilization or radiation therapy may be needed.

Visceral Pain

Visceral pain presumably results from activation of nociceptors in the viscera by compression, obstruction, infiltration, ischemia, stretching, or inflammation. When injury involves a hollow viscus, the pain usually is not well localized and often is described as cramping, gnawing, squeezing, or pressure. Depending on the structures involved, the pain may improve or worsen with eating or bowel movements or distension of the bladder or bowel. Injury to some visceral tissues, such as organ capsules, mesentery or other fascia, or the heart or pancreas, produces pain that is usually described as sharp or stabbing, referring to well-described patterns of certain anatomic areas.

Neuropathic Pain

Neuropathic pain results from injury to peripheral or CNS structures. Although neuropathic pain may be sharp, aching, and familiar, some patients develop a phenomenology characterized by a painful dysesthesia such as burning, shooting, tingling, stabbing, scalding, and painful numbness. Other aberrant sensations that may accompany the pain and disturbances of sensation, such as allodynia (pain from light touch or mild pressure) or hyperalgesia (increased response to a noxious stimulus),[35] may be prominent. Examples of chronic neuropathic pain syndromes include postherpetic neuralgia, postsurgical painful mononeuropathies (eg, postmastectomy and post-thoracotomy pain syndromes), chemotherapy-induced painful polyneuropathy, malignant plexopathy, and phantom pain syndromes.

Syndrome recognition may guide additional clinical evaluation and treatment, clarify prognosis, allow preventative care, or offer reassurance to patients who have interpreted the pain as a certain indication of disease progression. Numerous nociceptive and neuropathic pain syndromes associated with cancer have been described in observational studies (**Table 3**).[36]

Table 3. Chronic Pain Syndromes[37]

RELATED TO TUMOR		
Nociceptive Syndromes: Somatic	*Tumor-related bone pain*	Multifocal bone pain
		Vertebral syndromes • Atlanto-axial destruction and odontoid fracture • C7-T1 syndrome • T12-L1 syndrome • Sacral syndrome (back pain secondary to spinal cord compression)
		Pain syndromes related to pelvis and hip • Pelvic metastases • Hip joint syndrome
		Base of skull metastases • Orbital syndrome • Parasellar syndrome • Middle cranial fossa syndrome • Jugular foramen syndrome • Occipital condyle syndrome • Clivus syndrome • Sphenoid sinus syndrome
	Tumor-related soft tissue pain	• Headache and facial pain • Ear and eye pain syndromes • Pleural pain
	Paraneoplastic pain syndromes	Muscle cramps
		Other • Hypertrophic pulmonary osteoarthropathy • Tumor-related gynecomastia • Paraneoplastic pemphigus • Paraneoplastic Raynaud's phenomenon
Nociceptive Syndromes: Visceral		Hepatic distention syndrome
		Midline retroperitoneal syndrome
		Chronic intestinal obstruction
		Peritoneal carcinomatosis
		Malignant perineal pain
		Adrenal pain syndrome
		Ureteric obstruction

continued

Table 3. Chronic Pain Syndromes[37] *continued*

RELATED TO TUMOR

Neuropathic Syndromes	Leptomeningeal metastases
	Painful cranial neuralgias
	Glossopharyngeal neuralgia
	Trigeminal neuralgia
	Malignant painful radiculopathy

	Plexopathies
	• Cervical plexopathy
	• Malignant brachial plexopathy
	• Malignant lumbosacral plexopathy
	   – Lower lumbosacral plexopathy
	   – Sacral plexopathy
	   – Panplexopathy
	   – Coccygeal plexopathy

	Painful peripheral mononeuropathies
	Paraneoplastic sensory neuropathy

RELATED TO TREATMENT

Chemotherapy	Painful peripheral neuropathy
	Raynaud's syndrome
	Bony complications of long-term steroids • Avascular (aseptic) necrosis of femoral or humeral head • Vertebral compression fractures
Radiation	Radiation-induced brachial plexopathy
	Chronic radiation myelopathy
	Chronic radiation enteritis and proctitis
	Lymphedema pain
	Burning perineum syndrome
	Osteoradionecrosis
Surgery	Postmastectomy pain syndrome
	Postradical neck dissection pain
	Postthoracotomy pain syndrome
	Postthoracotomy frozen shoulder
	Postsurgery pelvic floor pain
	Stump pain
	Phantom pain

From Treatment of cancer pain, by RK Portenoy, 2011, Lancet, 377(9784), 2236-2247. © 2011 by Elsevier. Reprinted with permission.

Patient Assessment

Objectives of Pain Assessment

A competent pain assessment should be considered a standard of care.[11] It should provide the information necessary to develop a plan of care for pain management and also should elucidate other concerns that may influence the broader plan to address factors contributing to suffering and illness burden (**Table 4**). The pain assessment should determine the need for additional evaluation such as laboratory testing or diagnostic imaging that may be needed to define the etiology or pathophysiology of the pain, clarify the extent of disease, or assess clinical comorbidities. Based on the assessment, a plan of care for pain management may recommend disease-modifying therapy and one or more types of symptomatic treatments, usually beginning with pharmacotherapy. The concurrent plan may focus on other symptoms; the need for improved communication, goal setting, care coordination, concrete services, or family support; or on any of the other elements subsumed under a palliative plan of care. Over time, pain reassessments will revisit these varied recommendations.

Components of Pain Assessment

A thorough pain assessment includes a comprehensive history, physical examination, and review of diagnostic information (Table 4). History taking should employ empathetic listening and fully characterize each pain complaint. Standardized pain assessment tools can be used to record the characteristics of the pain and its impact on cognitive function, mood, sleep, appetite, physical activities, social functioning, and

---

Table 4. Key Objectives of a Pain Assessment[37]

1. To characterize the multiple dimensions of the pain (eg, using the "PQRST" mnemonic—see Table 5)
2. To formulate an understanding of the nature of the pain
   - Etiology
   - Inferred pathophysiology
   - Pain syndrome
3. To characterize the impact of the pain on quality-of-life domains
   - Effect on physical functioning and well-being
   - Effect on mood, coping, and related aspects of psychological well-being
   - Effect on role functioning and social and familial relationships
   - Effect on sleep, mood, vitality, and sexual function
4. To clarify the extent of the underlying disease, planned treatment, and prognosis
5. To clarify the nature and quality of prior testing and past treatments
6. To elucidate medical comorbidities
7. To elucidate psychiatric comorbidities
   - Substance use history
   - Depression and anxiety disorders
   - Personality disorders
8. To determine other needs for palliative care interventions
   - Other symptoms
   - Distress related to psychosocial or spiritual concerns
   - Caregiver burden and concrete needs
   - Problems in communication, care coordination, and goal setting

From Treatment of cancer pain, by RK Portenoy, 2011, Lancet, 377(9784), 2236-2247. © 2011 by Elsevier. Reprinted with permission.

overall quality of life, but, with the exception of a simple scale for pain severity, most clinicians rely in practice on the clinical history of these details.

The clinician may use the PQRST mnemonic to assist in characterizing the pain complaint (**Table 5**). Pain severity (the "S" in the mnemonic) may be measured using a simple verbal rating scale (eg, *mild*, *moderate*, *severe*) or some other unidimensional scale (**Figure 1**).[39] A numeric scale (eg, "on a scale from 0 to 10, where *0* equals no pain and *10* equals the worst possible pain, how severe is your pain right now?") may be administered verbally or in writing. Other scales such as the Visual Analog Scale (VAS) or a pictorial scale (eg, the Wong-Baker FACES™ Pain Rating Scale, developed specifically for children [**Figure 2**][40] or the Pain Thermometer[41,42]) are administered using a written tool. Patients representing a variety of cultures may find it easier to respond to individualized symbols for pain such as a series of pictures of fires that become increasingly larger. Older adults may prefer using pain terminology such as *discomfort*, *aching*, *hurting*, or *soreness* when using a pain scale. Regardless of which scale is used, it is important to continue using the same scale and terminology with the patient to ensure reliability.

The key requirements of pain measurement include the following:

1. Use the same tool repeatedly.
2. If possible, have the same clinician take the measurement each time.

3. When the measurement is taken, stipulate the intensity context and the time frame (eg, "pain right now," "pain on average during the past day," "pain at its worst during the past day," or "pain at its least during the past day") and consider asking about more than one descriptor (eg, "pain on average during the past day" and "pain at its worst during the past day").

Pain Assessment Scales

Multidimensional pain scales such as the McGill Pain Questionnaire (MPQ) and the Brief Pain Inventory (BPI) assess pain severity and other pain characteristics.[43] The MPQ evaluates pain qualities and the BPI focuses on pain's influence on mood and function. These instruments are seldom used in clinical practice in their entirety and are reserved for research.[43] The lengthier tools require patients to have fairly sophisticated language skills, and these tools may fatigue frail patients in the palliative care setting.

When patients are unable to communicate, behavioral observations substitute for self-report of pain intensity. Behaviors that may be interpreted as pain or distress include moaning, grimacing, and guarding. Many behavioral instruments have been validated for use in patients with severe cognitive impairment (see *UNIPAC 9*).

Assessing pain in the intensive care unit (ICU) can be challenging. Two pain behavior

---

Table 5. PQRST Pain Assessment Mnemonic[27]

P	Palliative, provocative factors: What makes the pain better or worse?
Q	Quality (word descriptors such as "burning" or "stabbing")
R	Region, radiation, referral (radicular, nonradicular pattern): Where does it hurt? Does the pain move or travel?
S	Severity (pain intensity rating scales or word descriptors)
T	Temporal factors (onset, duration, daily fluctuations): When did it start? Is it constant and/or intermittent? How long does it last? Is it better or worse at certain times of the day?

From Nonmalignant pain in palliative medicine (p. 934), by S Weinstein, in D Walsh, R Fainsinger, K Foley, et al. (Eds.), Palliative Medicine, 2009, Philadelphia: Saunders. © 2009 by Elsevier. Reprinted with permission.

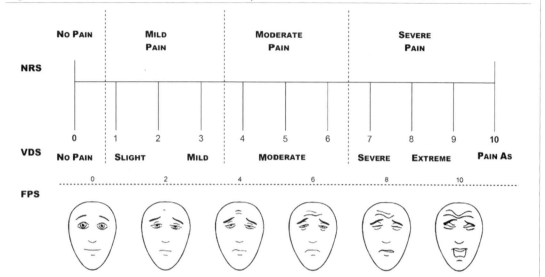

Figure 1. Unidimensional Pain Scales Compared with the Faces Pain Scale

FPS, Faces Pain Scale; NRS, numeric rating scale; VDS, verbal descriptor scale.

FPS instructions: When giving the following instructions, say "hurt" or "pain," whichever seems right for a particular child. "These faces show how much something can hurt. This face (point to left-most face) shows no pain. The faces show more and more pain (point to each from left to right) up to this one (point to right-most face)—it shows very much pain. Point to the face that shows how much you hurt (right now)." Score the chosen face 0, 2, 4, 6, 8, or 10, counting left to right so 0 = no pain and 10 = very much pain. Do not use words such as "happy" and "sad." This scale is intended to measure how children feel inside, not how their face looks.

From The Faces Pain Scale–Revised: toward a common metric in pediatric pain measurement, by CL Hicks, CL von Baeyer, P Spafford, I van Korlaar, and B Goodenough, 2001, Pain, 93, 173-183. The Faces Pain Scale for the self-assessment of the severity of pain experienced by children: development, initial validation and preliminary investigation for ratio scale properties, by D Bieri, R Reeve, GD Champion, L Addicoat, and J Ziegler, 1990, Pain, 41, 139-150. © 2001 by the International Association for the Study of Pain. Reprinted with permission.

Figure 2. Wong-Baker FACES™ Pain Rating Scale

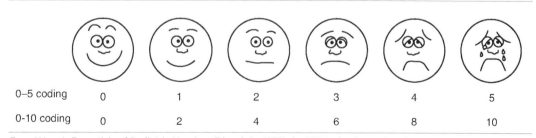

| 0–5 coding | 0 | 1 | 2 | 3 | 4 | 5 |
| 0-10 coding | 0 | 2 | 4 | 6 | 8 | 10 |

From Wong's Essentials of Pediatric Nursing, 7th ed. (p. 1259), by MJ Hockenberry, D Wilson, and ML Winkelstein, 2005, 1259. St. Louis: Mosby. © 2005 by Mosby. Reprinted with permission.

instruments have been tested for their reliability, validity, and feasibility of use in ICUs: the Pain Behavior Scale and the Critical-Care Pain Observation Tool.[44] Other tools include the pain assessment, intervention, and notation (PAIN) algorithm and a pain behaviors checklist.[45] According to Puntillo and colleagues, when established tools are insufficient to evaluate a patient's pain, alternative methods to augment a pain evaluation should be considered. These methods can include completing a pain risk profile using surrogates or performing an analgesic trial.[46] When working with deeply sedated patients in the ICU, neither verbal nor behavioral measures are feasible; in these cases physiologic changes, such as tachycardia and hypertension, may be used to track the potential effects of noxious stimuli.

In characterizing the pain complaint, temporal features must be explored (the "T" in the PQRST mnemonic). Most patients with advanced illness have constant or background pain with episodes of breakthrough pain. Accordingly, daily pain fluctuations superimposed on constant pain should be specifically evaluated. When asking about breakthrough pain, details related to frequency, onset, duration, predictability, and impact may be essential for deciding among the various treatment strategies for this component.

History Assessment

As part of the clinical history, the pain description should be supplemented with information about prior evaluation of the pain, prior treatment, and the impact of pain on various domains of function. A psychosocial assessment should be performed, both to assess the meaning of pain for the patient and family and to determine if other issues deserve attention in the broader plan of palliative care. The expression of pain is influenced by a patient's previous experience, culture, social milieu, personality, and situational stressors. Exploring the pain or other stressors

may reveal clues about the patient's usual coping strategies and resiliency, which in turn may influence therapeutic decisions. Clinicians also should elicit a history of chronic noncancer pain if present, and understand how the patient adapted to it.

Given the reliance on opioid therapy as a key approach to the treatment of pain in medically ill patients, it is extremely important to ask about the patient's previous and current relationships with potentially abusable drugs, including alcohol, controlled prescription drugs, and illicit drugs. When the family history is queried, it is equally important to determine whether drug abuse has occurred in the immediate family.

Patient Expectations and Goals

Clinicians must also ascertain the patient's and family's knowledge of expectations and goals for pain management when determining appropriate therapy. Patients with life-threatening illness frequently harbor anxieties and fears but may be reluctant to discuss them because of concerns that their thoughts and feelings will be considered strange or abnormal. To position pain management in the broader strategy for palliative care, clinicians should ask and listen for clues about the presence of psychological, social, and spiritual issues that may be contributing to suffering and amplifying the pain experience. By providing a nonjudgmental and compassionate presence, physicians and other members of the care team can provide therapeutic support that is always valuable and is sometimes more beneficial than additional tests or medical interventions.

Patient Concerns

When assessing the complex contributors to the suffering and illness burden experienced by patients and their families, it is useful to include open-ended questions during history taking. However, patients with severe physical pain may have limited ability to engage and, in such cases, lengthier discussion should be pursued only after the highest level of comfort is achieved. Examples of questions that may either illuminate the pain complaint or elicit concerns other than pain include the following:

- When people become seriously ill, they usually find themselves wondering why it happened to them. When you think about this, what comes to mind?
- When you think about the next few weeks or months, what are some concerns that first come to mind? What things concern you more than others?
- When you think back over the years, what are some of your happiest times? Saddest?
- What has given you strength in the past? What gives you strength now? What do you wish could happen to give you more strength?
- How has this illness affected you emotionally? What has been particularly difficult? Has anything been more (or less) difficult than you thought it might be?
- How is your family coping with this illness? Can you tell me something about what is going on with them? What are some of your concerns about your family?

The information acquired through this detailed history taking is necessary to establish working hypotheses about the nature of the pain and contextual information essential to optimize the plan of care. The next step, an examination, provides additional information about the pain itself and an assessment of the disease status, comorbidities, and the general physical condition of the patient[47] (**Table 6**).

Physical Examination

In many cases a physical examination begins with vital signs. But the physiological signs of acute pain such as elevated blood pressure, respiratory rate, and pulse are unreliable indicators of acute pain and typically disappear when pain persists. Patients commonly experience severe pain with entirely normal vital signs.

Table 6. Physical Examination[27]

General Inspection
- Patient's appearance and vital signs
- Evidence of abnormalities such as weight loss, muscle atrophy, deformities, trophic changes

Pain Site Assessment
- Inspect the pain sites for abnormal appearance or color of overlying skin, change of contour, or visible muscle spasm.
- Palpate the sites for tenderness and texture.
- Use percussion to elicit, reproduce, or evaluate the pain and any tenderness on palpation.
- Determine the effects of physical factors such as position, pressure, and motion.

Neurological Examination
- Mental status: level of alertness, higher cognitive functions, affect
- Cranial nerves
- Sensory system: light touch and pinprick test to assess for allodynia, evoked dysesthesia, hypesthesia/hyperesthesia, hypalgesia/hyperalgesia, hyperpathia
- Motor system: muscle bulk and tone, abnormal movements, manual motor testing, reflexes
- Coordination, station, and gait

Musculoskeletal Examination
- Body type, posture, and overall symmetry
- Abnormal spine curvature, limb alignment, and other deformities
- Range of motion (spine, extremities)
- For muscles in the neck, upper extremities, trunk, and lower extremities: Observe for any abnormalities such as atrophy, hypertrophy, irritability, tenderness, and trigger points.

From Nonmalignant pain in palliative medicine (p. 934), by S Weinstein, in D Walsh, R Fainsinger, K Foley, et al. (Eds.), Palliative Medicine, 2009, Philadelphia: Saunders. © 2009 by Elsevier. Reprinted with permission.

In most cases the examination should include both a neurological and musculoskeletal assessment. Pain associated with neurological findings may suggest neuropathic mechanisms; the absence of neurological findings, however, does not exclude this diagnosis. Pain that is reproduced by mechanical factors such as joint motion, weight bearing, or gait suggests an etiology involving the musculoskeletal system. In the soft tissues, one may palpate muscle spasms or discrete trigger points which, when stimulated, refer pain to another site.

Review of Data

The pain evaluation concludes with a review of available laboratory and imaging studies. When caring for imminently dying patients, further information of this type is not actionable and should be eschewed. At other times, however, the nature of the complaint and goals of care indicate the need for additional tests to establish the diagnosis of the pain, evaluate the extent of disease, and determine the feasibility of disease-modifying therapy (**Table 7**). In those with a history of chronic pain preceding the present illness, a critical evaluation of the history, findings on examination, and imaging studies may be necessary to determine whether the etiology of a painful disorder is related to the life-threatening illness.[48]

In some cases, changes in pain or associated manifestations over time may be necessary to clarify a differential diagnosis. This information may be obtained from a patient's history or a pain diary that helps establish the pattern of painful episodes.[49] For example, important information can be obtained from a diary kept by a patient with chronic headache who develops metastatic disease. Stable recurrent episodes of headache do not require repeated evaluation, but a change in headache pattern may call for reimaging or examination of the cerebrospinal fluid. In a similar way, the assessment and management of low back pain, joint pain, neuropathic pain states (eg, painful diabetic neuropathy, postherpetic neuralgia, nerve-injury related),[50,51] and other conditions such as fibromyalgia may require ongoing assessment of the pain pattern in the context of management strategies offered concurrently with treatments for the new illness.

Table 7. Diagnostic Testing for Pain[27]

Types of Tests	Uses
Screening laboratory tests: CBC, chemistry profile (eg, electrolytes, liver, enzymes, BUN, creatinine), urinalysis, ESR	Screen for medical illnesses, organ dysfunction
Disease-specific laboratory tests (includes autoantibodies, sickle cell test)	Autoimmune disorders, SCD
Imaging studies: radiographs, CT, MRI, US, myelography	Detection of tumors, other structural abnormalities
Diagnostic procedures: lumbar puncture for CSF analysis	Detection of various CNS illnesses
Electrophysiologic tests: EMG (direct examination of skeletal muscle), NCV (examination of conduction along peripheral nerves)	Detection of myopathy, neuropathy, radiculopathy
Diagnostic nerve block: injection of a local anesthetic to determine the source and mechanism of the pain	Identification of structures responsible for the pain (eg, sacroiliac or facet joint blocks), differentiation of pain pathophysiology

BUN, blood urea nitrogen; CBC, complete blood count; CNS, central nervous system; CSF, cerebrospinal fluid; CT, computed tomography; EMG, electromyography; ESR, erythrocyte sedimentation rate; MRI, magnetic resonance imaging; MS, multiple sclerosis; NCS, nerve conduction studies; NCV, nerve conduction velocity; SCD, sickle cell disease; US, ultrasound.

From Nonmalignant pain in palliative medicine (p. 934), by S Weinstein, in D Walsh, R Fainsinger, K Foley, et al. (Eds.), Palliative Medicine, *2009, Philadelphia: Saunders. © 2009 by Elsevier. Reprinted with permission.*

Pain Management

Treating chronic pain in patients with serious or life-threatening illness must be individualized, and the benefits and burdens related to the broader goals of palliative care must be balanced. If a patient has access to a specialist palliative care team, referral usually is considered when pain is difficult to control, is accompanied by other complex concerns, or occurs in the setting of far-advanced illness and short prognosis (the terminal care setting).[21] Some systems also have pain specialists, and patients with refractory pain may be able to access their expertise, as well.

Approach to Pain Management

Most pain can be managed with relatively simple approaches, however, when pain is difficult to control management may require complex pharmacotherapy or adjunctive strategies. The latter approaches include a large number of invasive treatments, which are generically labeled pain interventions.

Treatment Considerations

The first step in developing a treatment strategy is to consider the feasibility, appropriateness, and potential effects of primary disease-modifying therapy. For example, in the setting of cancer pain, radiotherapy is commonly administered for analgesia and may be highly effective, particularly in bone lesions.[52] Although the literature on the potential pain-relieving effects of chemotherapy is complicated by methodological issues, the large number of regimens used, the limited availability of comparative trials, and other concerns,[53,54] the potential for pain-relieving effects may be one factor considered in decisions about the use of chemotherapy. Similarly, cancer surgery also may have analgesic consequences, and

although pain is rarely the primary indication for an operation, it may be an important factor to consider. Palliative care clinicians should have a thorough understanding of the potential analgesic benefit of primary disease-modifying treatments for cancer and other serious illnesses.

Even if primary disease-modifying therapy is applied, most patients with persistent moderate or severe pain will require primary analgesic strategies. Pharmacotherapy is widely accepted as the main approach in the treatment of pain related to active, serious illness. Other approaches are considered when drug therapy does not promptly yield a satisfactory result (**Table 8**).

Pharmacologic Treatment

There are three main categories of drugs used to treat pain: the nonopioid analgesics, which in the United States include nonsteroidal anti-inflammatory drugs (NSAIDs) and acetaminophen; opioids; and an assortment of drug classes and agents referred to as adjuvant analgesics. Combination therapy is common in the treatment of chronic pain.

WHO Analgesic Ladder

Opioid-based pharmacotherapy has been viewed as the most important analgesic strategy for patients with life-threatening illness since the World Health Organization (WHO) posited the analgesic ladder approach for cancer pain more than 25 years ago (**Figure 3**).[5] The analgesic ladder is a simple framework for drug selection that incorporates guidelines for dose titration and other key aspects of treatment with opioids; surveys suggest the approach can be used to provide effective pain relief for up to 90% of patients.[5]

The original analgesic ladder framework recommended a nonopoid for mild pain, a so-called weak opioid for moderate pain, and a so-called strong opioid for severe pain (Figure 3). During the years since this approach was developed, the terms *weak* and *strong* have fallen out of favor. A variety of alternative strategies have been advanced to accomplish the fundamental goals of selecting analgesic therapy with regard for the severity of the pain to optimize dosing, manage side effects, and appropriately change therapy based on results. A broader modification of the approach to drug selection and dosing includes the following:

- Step 1. When pain is relatively mild, it may be sufficient to start with acetaminophen, an NSAID, or an adjuvant analgesic targeting a specific type of pain (eg, neuropathic, bone pain).

- Step 2. When pain persists, increases, or presents as mild to moderate, an opioid regimen should be considered. The choice may be an opioid used conventionally for moderate pain such as hydrocodone or codeine, a mixed-mechanism opioid (eg, tramadol, tapentadol), or a low starting dose of an opioid used conventionally for severe pain such as oxycodone or morphine. At Step 2, fixed-dosage combinations of an opioid with acetaminophen often are used because combining the drugs sometimes provides added analgesia. When higher dosages of an opioid are needed, single-entity opioid and nonopioids are used to avoid toxic effects of high-dose acetaminophen and other NSAIDs. Adjuvant analgesics also are considered for specific types of pain. When Step 2 is initiated, medications for persistent pain are administered on an around-the-clock basis, with additional dosages as needed to control breakthrough pain.

- Step 3. When pain persists, increases, or initially presents as moderate to severe, single-entity, pure mu-agonist opioids are administered (eg, morphine, oxycodone, oxymorphone, hydromorphone, methadone, or fentanyl). Again, treatment usually involves around-the-clock administration for persistent pain, plus a supplemental short-acting drug as-needed for breakthrough pain. Coadministration of acetaminophen, an NSAID, or an adjuvant analgesic may be considered.

Category	Type of Treatment
Pharmacological	Opioid analgesics
	Nonopioid analgesics
	Nontraditional analgesics ("adjuvant analgesics")
Interventional	Injection therapies
	Neural blockade
	Implant therapy
	Surgical neuroablation
Rehabilitative	Physical modalities such as ultrasound
	Therapeutic exercise
	Occupational therapy
	Hydrotherapy
	Therapy for specific disorders such as lymphedema
Psychological	Psychoeducational interventions
	Cognitive-behavioral therapy
	Relaxation therapy, guided imagery, other types of stress management
	Hypnotherapy
	Other forms of psychotherapy
Neurostimulation	Transcutaneous
	Transcranial
	Implanted
Complementary/ Alternative or Integrative	Acupuncture
	Massage
	Physical/movement
	Music therapy
	Art therapy
	Other

Table 8. Pain Treatment Categories[37]

From Treatment of cancer pain, by RK Portenoy, 2011, Lancet, 377(9784), 2236-2247. © 2011 by Elsevier. Reprinted with permission.

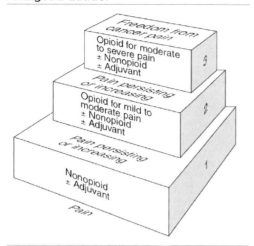
Opioid Analgesics

The goal of long-term treatment with opioid analgesics is to provide sustained, clinically meaningful relief of pain with side effects that are tolerable and an overall benefit to quality of life. Guidelines, which are based on extensive international experience, limited evidence, and expert review,[5,10-13,55] provide a rationale for the selection of drug and route of administration, dosing, and side-effect management.

Drug Selection

Pure mu-agonist opioids are conventionally selected for pain treatment (**Table 9**). Important exceptions are meperidine and propoxyphene (no longer available in the United States), which are not recommended because of their potential for adverse effects. Centrally acting drugs with mixed opioid-monoaminergic mechanisms such as tramadol and tapentadol may be used but have a ceiling due to risks at higher doses; consequently, they offer less dosing flexibility.

Although buprenorphine, a partial mu-receptor agonist and kappa-receptor antagonist, may also be used, pure mu-agonist drugs are preferred because experience with these drugs in medically ill patients is much more extensive. The mixed agonist-antagonist opioids such as pentazocine and butorphanol offer no advantage and also are not preferred in this setting.

Codeine and morphine were selected for the original WHO analgesic ladder, but there is no pharmacological rationale for this preference, particularly given the genetically determined variation in codeine's effects[56] and the potential influence of morphine metabolites in patients with renal impairment.[57] Experience with sequential opioid trials, or *opioid rotation*, highlights the importance of individual differences in response to various opioid drugs[58,59] and suggests that the most favorable opioid for an individual cannot be predicted. The important principle is that therapy may be initiated with any of the commonly used pure mu-agonist drugs, and clinicians should be prepared to switch, if necessary, to determine the drug that provides the best therapeutic outcomes.

The WHO analgesic ladder approach selects different opioids based on a moderate (eg, codeine) or severe (eg, morphine) pain intensity.[5] Although it remains common practice to follow this recommendation, any of the single-entity, pure mu-agonist drugs can be prescribed at doses low enough to safely manage moderate pain, which eliminates the second "rung" of the ladder.[60]

Regular administration of an opioid to prevent or minimize chronic pain can be accomplished with a short- or long-acting opioid. In developed countries, long-acting drugs—either modified-release formulations (which have dosing intervals of 8 hours to 3 days) or a drug with a half-life such as methadone—are generally viewed as advantageous. They may increase convenience, reduce

Table 9. Equianalgesic Table for Adults

MEDICATION	EQUIANALGESIC DOSE (for chronic dosing) SC/IV	EQUIANALGESIC DOSE (for chronic dosing) PO		USUAL STARTING DOSES Adult > 50 kg; for opioid-naïve patients (♦1/2 dose for elderly, or severe renal or liver disease) PARENTERAL	USUAL STARTING DOSES PO
MORPHINE	10 mg	30 mg		2.5-5 mg SC/IV q3-4h (♦1.25–2.5 mg)	5-15 mg q3-4h (IR or oral solution) (♦2.5-7.5 mg)
OXYCODONE	Not available	20 mg		Not available	5-10 mg q3-4h (♦2.5 mg)
HYDROMORPHONE	1.5 mg	7.5 mg		0.2-0.6 mg SC/IV q2-3h (♦0.2 mg)	1-2 mg q3-4h (♦0.5-1 mg)
CODEINE	130 mg	200 mg		15-30 mg IM/SC q4h (♦7.5-15 mg) IV Contraindicated	30-60 mg q3-4h (♦15-30 mg)
HYDROCODONE	Not available	30 mg		Not available	5 mg q3-4h (♦2.5 mg)
METHADONE (see text for dosing conversions)	½ oral dose 2 mg PO methadone = 1 mg parenteral methadone	24-hour oral morphine < 30 mg 31-99 mg 100-299 mg 300-499 mg 500-999 mg 1,000-1,200 mg > 1,200 mg	Oral morphine: methadone ratio 2:1 4:1 8:1 12:1 15:1 20:1 Consider consult	1.25-2.5 mg q8h (♦1.25 mg)	2.5-5 mg q8h (♦1.25-2.5 mg)
FENTANYL (see text for dosing conversions)	100 mcg single dose (T½ and duration of parenteral doses variable)	24-hr oral MS dose 30-59 mg 60-134 mg 135-224 mg 225-314 mg 315-404 mg	Initial patch dose 12.5 mcg/hr 25 mcg/hr 50 mcg/hr 75 mcg/hr 100 mcg/hr	25-50 mcg IM/IV q1-3h (♦12.5-25 mcg)	Transdermal patch 12.5 mcg/hr q72h (Use with caution in opioid-naïve and unstable patients because of 12-hour delay in onset and offset)

NOT RECOMMENDED

MEDICATION	SC/IV	PO		PARENTERAL	PO
MEPERIDINE	75-100 mg	300 mg		75 mg SC/IM q2-3h (♦25-50 mg) Generally not recommended	Not recommended

Developed by palliative care programs at University of Rochester Medical Center, ViaHealth, Unity Health, and Excellus BlueCross/BlueShield. Adapted from Guide to Alleviating Physical and Psychological Pain in Patients with Serious or Life-Threatening Conditions. © 2012 by Timothy E. Quill. *Adapted with permission.*

continued

Table 9. Equianalgesic Table for Adults *continued*

Fentanyl and Methadone: Special Considerations

Expert panels designated transdermal (TD) fentanyl and methadone as exceptions to the 30%-50% equianalgesic dosage reduction to account for incomplete cross-tolerance, and each poses distinct challenges for dosing in general.[1,2]

Fentanyl

- Conversion ratios from oral morphine to TD fentanyl shown in the table include a correction factor for incomplete cross-tolerance; routine 30% reduction of the equianalgesic amount is likely unnecessary.
- When converting from TD fentanyl to oral morphine, use the most conservative end of the range (ie, 50% rather than 30% reduction).
- TD fentanyl is stored in fat cells and then gradually released; it takes 12-24 hours to take full effect and 12-24 hours to dissipate once removed, which makes it easy to manage once a steady state is achieved (it will usually last 72 hours between patches), but it is very difficult to use for pain that is changing rapidly.
- Release of TD fentanyl from the patch may be accelerated if the patient becomes febrile.
- Dosing the new transmucosal fentanyl preparations should always start at the lowest available dosage regardless of the baseline regimen.[1]

Note. Rules for prescribing transmucosal fentanyl as a breakthrough medication should not be considered the same as for other opioids in terms of the ratio between the total daily dosage and the breakthrough dose. Immediate release oral and buccal fentanyl preparations are expensive and have unique properties with which prescribers should become familiar before prescribing. Usually other short-acting opioids are preferable for breakthrough prescribing when using TD fentanyl as a baseline medication.

Methadone

- Methadone has a long, variable half-life (ranging from 6-190 hours). The rapid titration guidelines used for other opioids do not apply to methadone. Dose-conversion ratios are complex and vary based on current opioid dosage and individual factors (see table).
- Because of the potential for drug accumulation from the long half-life, always write "hold for sedation" when initially prescribing or changing dosages of methadone.
- Methadone is better used as a baseline, scheduled analgesic, with shorter-acting opioids such as morphine or hydromorphone used prn. In stable situations, small doses of methadone can be given prn in addition to the scheduled regimen, but never more than 2.5 mg-5 mg two or three times daily. Small incremental doses in patients receiving a large baseline dose may have a major effect on blood level if taken regularly.
- When converting from oral to IV methadone, reduce the total daily dose of methadone by 50%.
- When converting from IV methadone to oral methadone, use 1 : 1 conversion to avoid overmedicating the patient; carefully observe the patient for under- and overdosing.

Note. Under most circumstances it is safer to use a different opioid with a much shorter half-life prn when using methadone as the baseline opioid. The usual calculation ratios and intervals used for determining breakthrough doses of other opioids do not apply to methadone (and fentanyl).

Cautions About Methadone

- The long half-life can lead to drug accumulation, sedation, confusion, and respiratory depression, especially in the elderly or with rapid dose adjustments.
- Methadone in moderate to high dosages can prolong the QTc interval and increase the risk of the potentially lethal *torsades de pointes* arrhythmia.[3] Depending on goals of treatment, presence of associated heart disease, patient's prognosis, presence of other medications that might cause similar problems (eg, haloperidol), or presence of new QTc prolongation risk factors, consider checking the QTc at baseline, and begin monitoring after each dose change for patients taking more than 100 mg of methadone daily. If QTc becomes significantly prolonged (450-499 ms = moderate risk; > 500 ms = high risk), consider lowering the methadone dose or rotate to an alternate opioid. Consider formal consultation with palliative care, acute pain service, cardiology, and pharmacy.
- Medications that can decrease methadone levels include rifampin, phenytoin, corticosteroids, carbamazepime, bosentan, phenobarbital, St. John's Wort, and a number of antiretroviral agents.
- Medications that can increase methadone levels include tricyclic antidepressants, azole antifungals (especially voriconazole), macrolides and fluoroquinolones, amiodarone, SSRIs, and diazepam. Grapefruit juice also can increase methadone levels.

References

1. Fine PG, Portenoy RK. Establishing "best practices" for opioid rotation: conclusions of an expert panel. *J Pain Symptom Manage.* 2009;38(3):418-425.
2. Knotkova H, Fine PG, Portenoy RK. Opioid rotation: the science and the limitations of the equianalgesic dose table. *J Pain Symptom Manage.* 2009;38(3):426-439.
3. Krantz MJ, Martin J, Stimmel B, Mehta D, Haigney MCP. QTc interval screening in methadone treatment. *Ann Int Med.* 2009;150:1-9.

continued

Table 9. Equianalgesic Table for Adults *continued*

Guidelines and principles are intended to be flexible. They serve as reference points or recommendations, not rigid criteria. Guidelines and principles should be followed in most cases, but there is an understanding that, depending on the patient, the setting, the circumstances, or other factors, care can and should be tailored to fit individual needs. (Revised 12/2009)

Guidelines*
1. Evaluate pain on all patients using a 0–10 scale.
   A. Mild pain: 1–3
   B. Moderate pain: 4–6
   C. Severe pain: 7–10
2. For chronic moderate or severe pain:
   A. Give baseline medication around the clock.
   B. Order 10% total daily dose as a prn given every 1-2 hours for oral and every 30-60 minutes for SC/IV.
   C. For continuous infusion, prn can be either the hourly rate every 15 minutes or 10% of total daily dose every 30-60 minutes.
   D. Adjust baseline upward daily in amount roughly equivalent to total amount of prn.
   E. Negotiate with patient target level of relief, but usually at least achieving level < 4.
3. In general, oral route is preferable, then transcutaneous > subcutaneous > intravenous.
4. When converting from one opioid to another, some experts recommend reducing the equianalgesic dose by ⅓ to ½, then titrate as in #2 above. Switching to methadone or to transdermal fentanyl are exceptions to this guideline.
5. Elderly patients, or those with severe renal or liver disease, should start on half the usual starting dose.
6. If parenteral medication is needed for mild to moderate pain, use half the usual starting dose of morphine or equivalent.
7. Refer to PDR for additional fentanyl guidelines.
8. Naloxone (Narcan) should only be used in emergencies:
   - Dilute naloxone 0.4 mg with 9 ml NS.
   - Give 0.1 mg (2.5 ml) slow IVP until effect.
   - Monitor patient every 15 minutes.
   - May need to repeat naloxone again in 30-60 minutes.
9. Short-acting preparations should be used acutely and postop. Switch to long-acting preparations when pain is chronic and the total daily dose is determined.

Information adapted from Drug Facts and Comparisons 2008, 62nd ed., by Facts & Comparisons, 2007, Philadelphia, PA: Lippincott Williams & Wilkins; and Principles of Analgesic Use in the Treatment of Acute Pain and Cancer Pain, 6th ed., by the American Pain Society, 2009, Glenview, IL: American Pain Society.

Developed by palliative care programs at University of Rochester Medical Center, ViaHealth, Unity Health, and Excellus BlueCross/BlueShield.

pill burden, and, at least theoretically, reduce the risk of a *bolus effect*—side effects at peak concentration or pain return at trough concentration. The ability to provide satisfactory relief with fixed-schedule dosages of a short-acting drug has been recognized for decades and remains an option in practice.

In the United States newer modified-release formulations such as long-acting oxycodone and morphine now include abuse-deterrent technology.[61] These formulations incorporate either a mechanical or chemical strategy to reduce the likelihood that a tablet can be converted into an immediate-release opioid by crushing or dissolving. The objective is to benefit the public health by reducing the likelihood of abuse and unintentional overdose and possibly decreasing street market value to mitigate diversion. These benefits have not been established empirically, and their effects on pain management remain unknown.

Drugs for Breakthrough Pain

Breakthrough pain has been reported in 40% to 80% of patients with cancer, depending on the clinical setting.[62,63] **Table 10** discusses different types of breakthrough pain. With growing recognition of the potential negative consequences resulting from breakthrough pain,[64]

Table 10. Types of Breakthrough Pain

Type	Characteristics	Pharmacologic Strategies
Incident	Activity-related Has identifiable precipitant	Use a short-acting rescue dose if possible; anticipate and premedicate with a short-acting agent; optimize the baseline regimen.
Idiopathic/ spontaneous	Unpredictable	Use a short-acting rescue dose if possible; optimize the baseline regimen.
End-of-dose failure	Predictable return of pain before next scheduled dose of medication	Increase the dose or shorten the time between doses of the baseline regimen or, if necessary, use a short-acting rescue dose.

a short-acting drug is usually offered as needed during regular opioid treatment. Depending on the dose required and other factors, this drug may be an opioid-nonopioid combination product, a single-entity oral opioid such as morphine or oxycodone, or a rapid-onset fentanyl formulation.

These supplemental opioid doses for breakthrough pain variably are called *rescue doses*, *breakthrough doses*, or *escape doses*. If an oral formulation is used, the dose usually is 5% to 15% of the baseline dose every 1 to 2 hours. For example, a patient receiving modified-release morphine at a dose of 100 mg every 12 hours (100 mg × 2 doses = 200 mg daily) may be prescribed a rescue dose of 10 mg to 30 mg every 1 to 2 hours. For patients receiving an opioid infusion, a dose equal to 50% to 100% of the hourly infusion rate every 10 to 15 minutes can be used. For example, a patient receiving a hydromorphone infusion at 1 mg/hour may be offered a rescue dose of 0.5 mg to 1 mg every 10 to 15 minutes. The safety of this proportionate dosing has not been established for rapid-onset fentanyl formulations, and treatment with these drugs should start with the lowest or next-to-lowest dose strength.[65]

In all cases titration of the rescue dose may be needed to optimize the balance between analgesia and side effects. If a rescue dose is needed three or more times daily, this may signal the need to increase the baseline dose or change the analgesic strategy.

The rapid-onset fentanyl formulations were developed to address the evident mismatch between the time course of typical breakthrough pain (most pains peak within minutes and last less than 1 hour) and the time-action relationship of an oral drug (onset is usually in 30 to 45 minutes and peak effects occur after 1 hour). All of these formulations, which now include an oral transmucosal lozenge, an effervescent buccal tablet, a buccal patch, a sublingual tablet, and nasal sprays, provide a means for a highly lipophilic drug to enter the bloodstream quickly via the transmucosal route. Clinical observations and limited comparative trials[66] suggest that the rapid-onset formulations yield faster pain relief and better outcomes, at least for some patients.[67,68] Although further study will be needed to assess the safety of these drugs and optimally position them relative to oral agents, it is reasonable to consider them for patients with severe breakthrough pain that peaks quickly, for those who do not respond well to oral drugs, and for patients lacking availability of the oral route.

Routes of Administration

The oral and transdermal routes of administration are preferred for long-term management of pain. The intramuscular route is not used because it is painful and provides no pharmacological advantage. Alternative routes of administration are considered in select circumstances.

Jimmy

Jimmy is a 45-year-old White male with laryngeal cancer who had major surgery, including resection and reconstruction. He is undergoing chemotherapy and radiation and has severe mouth and neck pain, along with mucositis. He is no longer able to swallow and receives all of his nutrition and medication through a percutaneous endoscopic gastrostomy (PEG) tube. His current pain management consists of oxycodone extended release (ER), 15 mg every 12 hours, with oxycodone, 5 mg for breakthrough pain. He currently crushes all of his medications and takes them through the PEG tube.

- What are the major problems you see in this case?
- What instructions would you give to this patient?
- Are there some alternative routes of administration that would be more appropriate?
- What pain regimen would you recommend?

Transdermal Administration

Although most clinicians consider the oral route first, some patients prefer transdermal administration, some benefit from access to fentanyl specifically, and some have problems with swallowing or gastrointestinal (GI) absorption that may be addressed through non-oral drug administration.[69] Several studies suggest the transdermal fentanyl formulation may yield less risk of constipation,[70] and this may be another reason to offer this route.

When initiating treatment with the transdermal fentanyl formulation, the equianalgesic dose table from the package insert may be used to select a starting dose (**Table 11**). The dose ratios built into this table are conservative, and most patients will require dose escalation to experience pain relief. A simple alternative method of initial dose selection is to divide the 24-hour total dose of oral morphine by 2 to get a starting dose of transdermal fentanyl.[71] For example, a patient taking 400 mg of oral morphine in 24 hours would be switched to 200 mcg/hour transdermal fentanyl every 72 hours.

Like other long-acting drugs, transdermal fentanyl should not be used to rapidly titrate the dose when pain is severe. In most situations the dose should not be titrated upward more frequently than every 72 hours. Because clinically relevant plasma fentanyl concentrations do not occur for 12 to 24 hours after the initial dose is applied, patients should be continued on their previous drugs for this period of time following a switch to transdermal fentanyl.[73] The coadministration of a short-acting rescue dose also provides a means to avoid uncontrolled pain during initial titration.

The risks associated with transdermal fentanyl are much like risks associated with all opioids, with a few exceptions. The most important difference is the risk of unintentional overdose from increased absorption associated with heat, either due to fever or an external heat source. As a result of this concern, the patch is not preferred in patients with recurrent fever.

Sublingual Administration

Occasionally, the sublingual route of administration is considered for patients who lose the ability to swallow. The lipophilic opioids such as fentanyl, methadone, and buprenorphine are absorbed through the oral mucosa relatively well.[74] Sublingual administration of the injectable fentanyl can be employed, if the dose required is relatively low; methadone may be considered

Table 11. Recommended Initial Transdermal Fentanyl Dose Based on Daily Oral Morphine Dose[72]

Oral 24-Hour Morphine (mg/day)	Transdermal Fentanyl Dose (mcg/hour)
60-134*	25
135-224	50
225-314	75
315-404	100

Pediatric patients initiating therapy on a 12 mcg/hour transdermal fentanyl system should be opioid tolerant and receiving at least 30-mg oral morphine equivalents per day (see UNIPAC 8).

as long as guidelines for safe administration are followed (see information about opioid rotation below), but sublingual buprenorphine can induce withdrawal if administered to patients who have been receiving another opioid. Consequently, it should only be used by knowledgeable clinicians experienced in its administration.

Other immediate-release oral formulations such as morphine, oxycodone, or hydromorphone are sometimes tried in the clinical setting; anecdotally, they appear to be adequate for some patients.[75,76] However, transmucosal absorption of these relatively hydrophilic drugs is minor and variable and most of the effects presumably relate to swallowed drug.

Rectal Administration

A variety of opioids and adjuvant medications can be administered rectally in suppository form. Slow-release morphine tablets inserted into an empty, moist rectum can deliver 12 hours of analgesia, comparable to their effect when given orally.[77] Custom-made methadone suppositories have proved effective in a wide range of dosages.[78,79] A number of adjuvant analgesics such as naproxen or valproic acid can be administered rectally by instilling the oral solution into the rectum using an enema bulb, urinary catheter, or a 6-inch length of nasal-prong oxygen tubing attached to a syringe. Some drugs such as doxepin come in gelatin capsules that dissolve in the rectum. Others can be crushed and put into large gel caps for rectal insertion.[80]

Rectal administration is associated with variable absorption because of variation in venous drainage, placement of the suppository, and contents of the rectum. Long-term administration in sentient patients is rarely acceptable. Accordingly, rectal administration is usually considered for short-term drug administration, perhaps in actively dying patients or as an interim step during the transition from oral to long-term parenteral administration.

Parenteral Administration

Patients who may benefit from long-term parenteral drug administration include those with dysphagia, persistent nausea and vomiting, delirium, or stupor. Patients receiving high dosages of oral medications that require numerous tablets are also good candidates. Long-term intravenous (IV) or subcutaneous (SC) drug administration may be provided as repeated boluses or infusions. With widespread access to syringe drivers (**Figure 4**) or other types of pumps in developed countries, infusions tend to be preferred.

Patients who have an indwelling central venous catheter have access for long-term IV therapy. The advent of peripherally inserted central catheters has expanded this opportunity. These catheters can be placed with minimal patient burden and low risk and may be used on a long-term basis.[81]

SC administration is a simple alternative to the IV route and can be accomplished using a butterfly catheter with a small-gauge needle inserted under the skin for 1 week or more. This catheter can be accessed for repeated boluses or connected to a pump for continuous SC infusion. Any opioid, or combination of opioid and adjuvant drug (eg, opioid plus antiemetic such as meta-clopramide or haloperidol) available in inject-able formulations can be administered in this way[82]; however, methadone can produce painful SC nodules during long-term SC dosing and is not preferred by this route. Morphine and hydro-morphone are the most common drugs selected for continuous infusion. Morphine can be used in dose strengths of up to 50 mg/mL, but because of its high solubility, hydromorphone is a better choice for high-dose infusions. Concentrated hydromorphone solution (10 mg/mL) is available, but if the doses required are high, more concen-trated solutions (eg, 50 mg/mL to 200 mg/mL) can be mixed from powder to avoid excess fluid administration during opioid infusion.

Hydration via the SC route (known as hypo-dermoclysis) is a well-known technique that can be combined with drug administration.

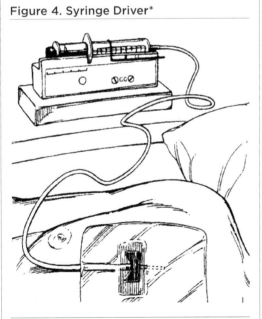

Figure 4. Syringe Driver*

*The skin over the outer deltoid or quadricep is less likely to cause a pneumothorax than is the skin over the pectoral area as illustrated above.

Hyaluronidase can be added to the infusate to facilitate high volume SC infusion.

For patients who are administered an oral opioid and switched to the IV or SC route using the same drug, the dose of the parenteral drug should be selected using the equianalgesic dose table (**Table 12**). It may be prudent to reduce the calculated dose by a small percentage because of variation in oral bioavailability. To calculate the required daily dosage of parenteral morphine, the patient's 24-hour oral morphine dose may be divided by 3, and this amount may be reduced by another 25%; the total divided by 24 is the hourly initial rate for a parenteral infusion (Table 12). Similar calculations are used for other drugs.

Patients receiving parenteral infusion for pain are usually offered a supplemental rescue dose for breakthrough pain. Pumps that have a patient-controlled analgesia (PCA) option are often used if the patient has the requisite cog-nitive and physical abilities needed to operate the device.[83] As described above, the rescue dose during parenteral infusion is usually proportional to the infused dose, either 5% to 15% of the total daily dose or more simply, 50% to 100% of the amount administered over a 1-hour period. This rescue dose can be offered every 10 to 15 minutes as needed. If more than three boluses are needed during the day, an increase in the baseline dose should be considered. Titration of the baseline dose more than once per day may be appropriate when the patient can be monitored and rescue doses are required frequently (eg, three or more doses in an 8-hour period).

Patients who are selected for repeated bolus therapy, rather than infusion, may simplify this approach with the use of a PCA device that is ordered without a basal infusion of opioids. This may be considered for patients who are relatively opioid naive and require rapid titration of a dose for more severe pain. The initial dose finding with

Table 12. Opioid Relative Potencies (Equianalgesic Doses)

Drug	Oral/Rectal (mg)	IV/SC (mg)
Morphine	30	10
Oxycodone	20	N/A
Hydromorphone	7.5	1.5
Hydrocodone	30	N/A
Oxymorphone	10	1
Fentanyl	N/A	100 mcg (single dose)

IV, intravenous; SC, subcutaneous.

the PCA alone may allow a more informed selection of the infusion rate after 1 to 2 days.

Neuraxial Drug Administration

Properly selected patients can benefit from spinal analgesic therapy, known generically as neuraxial infusion.[84] A randomized trial comparing conventional analgesic therapy and neuraxial infusion via an implanted programmable pump in patients with cancer found that neuraxial infusion yielded better analgesia and fewer side effects.[85] If this option exists, it should be considered among a range of strategies for patients with pain refractory to routine systemic therapy.

The best indication for a trial of neuraxial infusion exists when a patient experiences meaningful pain relief during systemic therapy with an opioid, but is unable to tolerate the side effects. In this situation many options may be considered, the most common of which presumably is opioid rotation. Neuraxial analgesia is another strategy.[86,87]

Neuraxial analgesia may be provided through either the epidural or subarachnoid (intrathecal) route. Epidural drug administration may be accomplished using a percutaneous catheter (either anchored to the back or tunneled SC and emerging anteriorly) or a catheter that is tunneled and connected to an implanted port. The former route is simpler to implement but less durable and more subject to infection or technical problems such as catheter dislodgement. For patients with a perceived life expectancy of more than 3 months and for those with pathology that complicates placement of an epidural catheter, such as vertebral compression fractures or radiation-induced fibrosis,[86] the intrathecal route is preferred. Based on limited data, it is generally accepted that the cumulative costs of an implanted system are lower than for an epidural system if the patient has a life expectancy of 3 months or longer.

The use of neuraxial analgesia requires strong collaboration with an interventional pain specialist. Follow-up care must be available for the patient, and the patient or family must be able to care for the catheter if it is externalized.[87] Competent clinical follow up must be available to address dosing issues or complications such as catheter occlusion, infection, and dislodgement.[88]

Robert

Robert is a 56-year-old African American male with severe chronic obstructive pulmonary disease, coronary artery disease, and lung cancer. He was initially diagnosed last year as stage IIIA and is undergoing chemotherapy. He is currently on oxycodone extended release, 10 mg every 12 hours, and occasionally takes a 5-mg oxycodone immediate-release tablet for breakthrough pain for his chronic chest pain.

He is admitted to the hospital with new onset back pain (10 on a 10-point scale) and dyspnea. He is found to have metastases in both lungs, pleural effusions, and multiple vertebral metastases. He is given 4 mg IV morphine in the emergency department with moderate effect on his back pain and is admitted to the hematology/oncology service. A palliative care team is called to assist with pain management only. When you enter the room, Robert is diaphoretic, tachypneic, grasping the bed rails, and crying out in pain. The nurse stops you at the door and asks if she can give him another 4-mg IV push of morphine since he tolerated it in the emergency department. Upon walking in the door, you see that Robert is in agony and respond to the nurse with "yes" as you proceed with the assessment.

Question One

Which of the following is most important in your initial pain assessment? (Choose all that apply.)

A. Explore Robert's emotional and spiritual concerns and how they may be affecting his pain.

B. Ask Robert to describe the pain—location, severity, quality, radiation, exacerbating and alleviating factors, and temporal factors—in his own words.

C. Perform a focused exam with special attention to the neurological exam.

D. Ask Robert about medications he has taken in the past that have helped and how the morphine he received in the emergency department affected his pain.

Correct Response and Analysis

Answers B, C, and D are all correct. It is important for the clinician to recognize a pain crisis and to obtain a focused history and physical exam.

Although A is important information to obtain, this is better done later outside of a crisis situation. A cancer patient with new or worsening back pain is at high risk for spinal cord compression, and recognizing this emergency is essential in guiding therapy.

The Case Continues

After two doses of 4-mg IV morphine, Robert reports that the pain improves from a 10 on a 10-point scale to an 8, but the effect only lasts about 30 minutes. He is not exhibiting any somnolence or altered mentation. He describes weakness in his legs and new dribbling after urination for the past 24 hours.

Question Two

What is the best initial approach to Robert's pain management? (Choose all that apply.)

A. Increase his oxycodone extended release to 20 mg every 12 hours and increase his oxycodone immediate release to 10 mg every 3 hours as needed.

B. Start scheduled high-dose IV steroids.

C. Give IV pushes of morphine with rapid titration every 30 minutes until pain is under better control.

D. Start ibuprofen by mouth as needed.

Correct Response and Analysis

B and C are correct in the setting of an acute pain crisis. Rapid titration of IV medications is the best initial approach.

A and D, although not harmful to the patient, would do very little for his pain in this setting. You have recognized the importance of ruling out a spinal cord compression, so a high-dose IV steroid, such as dexamethasone, would be an appropriate adjuvant medication, and since the patient tolerated IV morphine, increasing doses with rapid titration are the most important interventions initially.

Continued on page 34

Opioid Titration

Practical Considerations in Dose Titration

Individualization of the opioid dose is the key to optimizing the balance between pain relief and side effects. Dose titration usually is necessary after therapy is initiated and may be needed whenever pain worsens or improves as a result of the disease, its treatment, or other factors.

For constant or frequently recurrent pain, an opioid should be taken on a regular schedule. The schedule should be selected according to the known duration of analgesic action of the particular agent. Modified-release formulations are available for dosing at intervals of 12 or 24 hours, or in the case of the transdermal fentanyl patch, 2 to 3 days.

Starting Dosage

The appropriate starting dosage of an opioid depends on several factors, including the frequency and severity of pain, previous experience with opioid analgesics, recent exposure to opioids, age and body weight (especially for young children and frail elderly people), and medical status. When initiating therapy for opioid-naive adults with chronic pain, the safest approach is to start with a low dosage of a short-acting oral formulation such as 5 mg of hydrocodone (in a hydrocodone-acetaminophen combination product), 2.5 mg to 5 mg of oxycodone (in an oxycodone-acetaminophen combination product), 1 mg to 2 mg of hydromorphone, or 5 mg to 10 mg of morphine every 3 to 4 hours.

As an alternative, opioid-naive adults with moderate chronic pain can be started on a modified-release formulation at a very low dose. Modified-release oral hydromophone at a dose of 8 mg/day, and modified-release morphine at a dose of 15 mg twice daily or 20 mg to 30 mg once daily, are examples. However, if rapid dose titration will be needed the use of a long-acting drug is not preferred. If titration is performed with a short-acting drug, a switch to a modified-release product can be done when the dose begins to stabilize.

The initial opioid dose should be titrated upward until relief is achieved or side effects supervene. A supplemental rescue dose can be offered as needed even if the baseline dose is administered as a short-acting formulation. To titrate an opioid, the dose usually is increased by 25% to 50% each increment, and sometimes higher (as much as 100%) if pain is severe and the patient is medically stable. Alternatively, the dose can be increased by an amount equal to the average daily consumption of rescue doses for breakthrough pain during the previous few days.

Ideally, the interval between dose escalations should be long enough to allow steady state to be approached. This is 2 to 3 days for the modified-release oral formulations and 3 to 6 days for the transdermal patch. This interval is usually 5 to 7 days for methadone because of its long elimination half-life, but it can be much longer.

When pain is severe, however, more rapid dose escalation is needed. Severe pain may be treated with IV bolus injections at short intervals to eliminate the absorption delay that occurs after each dose. Although aggressive dosing achieves analgesic blood levels quickly, it carries the risk of delayed toxicity as levels continue to rise toward steady state after the dose stabilizes at a level that provides prompt relief. To avoid toxicity related to this "overshooting," monitoring is needed after rapid dose adjustments until steady state is approached; if delayed somnolence or other adverse effects occur, the dose should be adjusted downward.

The dose of a short-acting drug given for breakthrough pain also must be adjusted over time to maintain effects. As noted, clinical experience suggests that the dose should remain in the range of 5% to 15% of the total daily dose, or 50% to 100% of the hourly infusion rate. Exceptions are the rapid-onset fentanyl formulations, which have effects at doses that may not be proportional to the fixed schedule dose.[64] As noted earlier, it is prudent to begin treatment with rapid-onset drugs at one of the lowest available doses and then titrate based on clinical response.

There is no maximal or optimal dose of the pure mu-agonist drugs. The general rule is that doses should be titrated upward until acceptable analgesia occurs or intolerable side effects demonstrate poor responsiveness to the drug. Most patients require relatively low doses (< 200 mg/day of morphine or equivalent), but some stabilize over time at doses many times higher (equivalent to grams of morphine per day). As the dose is increased, particularly to relatively high levels, subtle toxicities, drug-related behaviors, and the burdens associated with the number of tablets or patches should be carefully reassessed. If problems are not evident, dose escalation should continue until there is a favorable balance between analgesic and side effects, regardless of dose.

Patients who develop treatment-limiting opioid side effects during dose titration are considered poorly responsive to the specific regimen. Some clinical characteristics such as age (< 60 years), neuropathic pain, and incidental pain predict poor responsiveness.[89] If poor responsiveness is demonstrated, another therapeutic strategy must be selected (**Table 13**). Opioid rotation is one of the most common approaches in this setting.[58]

Opioid Rotation

When patients experience intolerable side effects or persistent pain despite escalating dosages of opioids, physicians may consider switching to a different opioid medication. Using a conversion table, a physician can compare potencies across different modes of administration (eg, oral versus IV) and different types of opioids (see Table 9). These values provide a guide that helps clinicians select a safe and effective dose of the new drug. It is important to recognize that the equianalgesic doses stated on conversion tables are based on older, single-dose studies, and that subsequent

Table 13. Clinical Strategies to Address Poor Opioid Responsiveness[37]

Approach	Options
Identify a more effective opioid	Opioid rotation
Open the "therapeutic window"	More aggressive side effect management
Add a systemic or spinal coanalgesic to reduce the opioid requirement	Coadministered NSAID, nontraditional analgesic, or a trial of neuraxial analgesia
Add a nonpharmacologic approach to reduce the opioid requirement	Neural blockade, a neurostimulatory approach, or psychological or rehabilitative therapy

From Treatment of cancer pain, by RK Portenoy, 2011, Lancet, 377(9784), 2236-2247. © 2011 by Elsevier. Reprinted with permission.

studies have revealed wide variability in conversion ratios.[90] Consequently, the equianalgesic dose table should be used only as a general guide.

Newer guidelines for opioid rotation emphasize safety by incorporating a two-step process to select the starting dose of the new drug[59] (**Table 14**). The first step involves calculating the equianalgesic dose (Table 9), followed by reducing the calculated dose to account for incomplete cross-tolerance and individual variation; the second step involves additional dose adjustment based on clinical factors. For example, a patient who is experiencing poor pain control and mental clouding while taking long-acting oxycodone at a dose of 60 mg twice daily might be considered for a switch to an alternative drug. There are no data to inform the selection of this drug and the decision usually is based on availability, cost, convenience, and previous experience. If morphine is selected, the 120 mg/day of oxycodone is roughly equianalgesic to a 180 mg/day dose of morphine. If a reduction of 25% is applied, the daily dose would be 135 mg. If the patient is medically frail, this might be decreased a small amount (to 120 mg/day) and a long-acting morphine might then be started at a dose of 60 mg twice daily. A rescue dose can also be offered, such as short-acting morphine, 15 mg every 2 hours as needed.

The method of opioid rotation shown in Table 14 can also be applied to drugs that are administered by other routes. It is prudent to reduce the calculated equianalgesic dose even if the same drug is to be administered by a different route given interindividual variation in bioavailability that characterizes this class.

Methadone Rotation

Rotation to methadone raises specific challenges and deserves additional comment. Methadone-associated risk has been receiving increasing

---

Table 14. Guidelines for Opioid Rotation

Step 1
- Select the new drug based on prior experience, availability, cost, and other factors.
- Calculate the equianalgesic dose from the equianalgesic dose table (see Table 9).
- If switching to any opioid other than methadone or fentanyl, identify an automatic dose reduction window of 25% to 50% less than the calculated equianalgesic dose.
- If switching to methadone, the automatic dose reduction window is 75% to 90%; rarely convert to methadone at a dose higher than 100 mg/day.
- If switching to transdermal fentanyl, do not use an automatic dose reduction; use the calculated equianalgesic dose included in the package insert.
- Select a dose closer to the lower bound (25% reduction) or the upper bound (50% reduction) of the automatic dose reduction window on the basis of a judgment that the equianalgesic dose table is relatively more or less applicable to the characteristics of the regimen or patient.
- Select a dose closer to the upper bound if the patient is receiving a relatively high dose of the current opioid, is not Caucasian, or is elderly or medically frail.
- Select a dose closer to the lower bound if upper-bound criteria are not met and if being switched to a different route using the same drug.

Step 2
- Based on assessment of pain severity and other medical or psychosocial characteristics, increase or decrease the calculated dose by 15% to 30% to enhance the likelihood the initial dose will be effective, or, conversely, is unlikely to cause withdrawal or side effects.
- Assess response and titrate the dose of the new opioid regimen to optimize outcomes.
- If a supplemental dose is used as needed, calculate this dose at 5% to 15% of the total daily opioid dose and administer at an appropriate interval; transmucosal fentanyl formulations are exceptions and always should be initiated at one of the lower doses.

From Treatment of cancer pain, by RK Portenoy, 2011, Lancet, *377(9784), 2236-2247. © 2011 by Elsevier. Reprinted with permission.*

scrutiny in populations with chronic noncancer pain,[91] and the lessons learned should be translated to medically ill patients. As noted, methadone often is considered when a high dose of another opioid results in unacceptable side effects.[92] In addition to its opioid agonist activity, methadone blocks the N-methyl-D-aspartate receptor (NMDA), which may contribute to analgesia and reverse a component of opioid analgesic tolerance.[92] Presumably as a consequence, methadone has a poorly predictable potency when administered after another opioid has been taken; its potency generally will be much greater if started after relatively high doses of another opioid have been taken[55] (Table 9). The potential for enhanced and unpredictable potency after a switch from any other opioid to methadone poses risk for unintentional overdose and has justified the recommendation that rotation to methadone be accompanied by a large reduction in the calculated equianalgesic dose.[59] The half-life of methadone averages about 24 hours but is highly variable, ranging from half a day to almost 1 week. This variably imposes additional risk. With steady-state levels in blood approached after 5 to 6 half-lives, effects must be monitored for a relatively long period after the dose is changed to anticipate the relatively long period required to be at steady state.

Several additional potential risks are associated with methadone. Given its metabolism by the cytochrome P450 system, drug-drug interactions are possible, particularly with drugs metabolized by CYP3A4.[93] Equally important, it is now appreciated that methadone prolongs the QTc interval, and knowledge of the baseline QTc and monitoring as methadone doses are increased[94] may be needed to optimize safety, particularly in the setting of polypharmacy to address multiple disorders.[95,96]

In short, despite strong analgesic potential, good oral bioavailability (80%), and relatively stable kinetics in renal impairment,[97] methadone has both unique pharmacokinetic and pharmacodynamic characteristics that may increase risk and must be understood to provide safe and effective therapy.[98] The potential for highly favorable outcomes has been suggested in observational studies,[99] and although controlled trials have not been able to confirm this benefit,[100,101] continued reliance on methadone is likely given clinical experience, its long dosing interval, flexibility by multiple routes,[102] and low cost. Its concurrent use as a treatment for opioid craving in those with addiction also suggests that it may have value when patients with substance use disorders develop pain; if a patient has an active substance use disorder, however, the complexity of management may be best addressed with the help of a specialist in addiction medicine.

Given the risks associated with methadone, a 2009 consensus document suggested specific guidelines for rotation to this drug.[59] Specifically, a switch to methadone from another opioid should be accompanied by a large reduction in the calculated equianalgesic dose. A decrease of 75% to 90% has been recommended; reductions near the upper bound of this range should be used when the switch is in the context of high-dose prior therapy or when patients are medically frail. A second-step dose change of up to 15% can be considered thereafter to accommodate more risk (eg, a dose reduction if there is a coadministered benzodiazepine) or severe pain (a dose increase).

Additional precautions should be observed: Treatment with methadone should be preceded by review of a baseline QTc interval in most cases. An interval of 500 milliseconds or longer should be considered an absolute contraindication to methadone therapy, and an interval longer than 450 milliseconds should be considered a relative contraindication and prompt an effort to remove other contributing factors to QTc prolongation (eg, another drug), if possible. Unless the goals of care are such that monitoring is not appropriate, repeated electrocardiograms (ECGs) during dose escalation must be considered, although a prospective trial did not conclude this intervention was essential for patients with cancer.[94] Monitoring of a patient's reaction to methadone should be frequent after therapy is initiated or the dose is increased; monitoring should become routine only when clinical stability has suggested steady-state levels. Methadone's risk profile is such that it is best used cautiously when other sedating centrally acting drugs are being administered, particularly benzodiazepines. Combination with benzodiazepines has anecdotally been linked with an increased risk of opioid-induced sleep-disordered breathing.

Other strategies have been developed for safe conversion from other opioids to methadone. One approach systematically alters the ratio used to calculate the equianalgesic dose based on the dose of the previous drug (**Table 15**).[103] It should be noted, however, that this approach has been associated with the need to increase this calculated dose by 25% to 50% for the first 2 days to avoid underdosing.[104]

Another published method involves conversion to a calculated dose over 3 days (**Table 16**).

Managing Opioid Side Effects

Effective treatment of side effects increases the likelihood of a favorable response to opioids and is consistent with the broader goals of palliative care. Common adverse effects include constipation and GI-related symptoms (ie, nausea, pyrosis, anorexia, bloating) as well as somnolence, mental clouding, or confusion. There are many other potential side effects. Most clinicians appreciate the possibility of dry mouth, sweating, pruritus or urticaria, urinary retention, or myoclonus. Less well known are the effects of hypogonadism (ie, fatigue, depressed mood, sexual dysfunction, loss of muscle mass) and sleep-disordered

Table 16. A Method to Rotate Opioids to Oral or Rectal Methadone

Day 1
- Decrease the previous opioid dosage by one-third.
- Replace with 3% of the previous daily oral morphine equivalent dosage given as oral or rectal methadone every 8 hours (eg, a patient receiving 1,000 mg of oral morphine is switched to 660 mg of oral morphine and 30 mg per day of oral methadone, such as 10 mg PO or PR every 8 hours).

Day 2
- Decrease the previous opioid by another one-third if pain is controlled with rescue doses of a short-acting opioid.
- Increase the methadone dosage only if pain is moderate to severe.

Day 3
- Discontinue the final one-third of the previous opioid.
- For breakthrough pain, give the patient a rescue dose of about 10% of the daily methadone dose, PO or PR.
- Continue daily assessment of pain and dose titration until reaching an effective stable dose of methadone.

PO, by mouth; PR, per rectum.

From Role of methadone in the management of pain in cancer patients, by E Bruera and CM Neumann, 1999, Oncology, 13(9), 1275-1282, 1285-1288, 1291. © 1999 by Mary Ann Liebert, Inc., Publishers. Adapted with permission.

Table 15. Methadone Conversion from Morphine Equivalent[103]

Morphine Equivalent	Methadone : Morphine Ratio
< 100 mg	1 : 3
101 mg-300 mg	1 : 5
301 mg-600 mg	1 : 10
601 mg-800 mg	1 : 12
801 mg-1,000 mg	1 : 15
> 1,000 mg	1 : 20

Robert's Case Continues

After receiving 20-mg IV morphine over the past hour and a dose of 10 mg IV dexamethasone, Robert relaxes and reports his pain at a 5 out of 10. Based on his opioid use, you start morphine via patient-controlled analgesia (PCA) and schedule his IV steroids. Robert receives an MRI scan, which shows metastases at the second and third lumbar vertebrae with extension into the epidural space. The hematology/oncology team consults with neurosurgery and radiation oncology clinicians. The next day, Robert reports that his pain is about a 4 out of 10 and is much improved. He has used 95 mg IV morphine in the last 24 hours. His neurological status has improved and is back to baseline after the steroids were initiated. Because of his poor performance status and comorbidities, the specialists feel that he is a high-risk surgical candidate, and the patient opts for palliative radiation only. The nurse calls you because Robert is starting to have severe myoclonus. It is interfering with his ability to sleep and eat.

Question Three

What are the best options for manging opioid-induced myoclonus? (Choose all that apply.)

A. Rotate Robert's medication to another opioid, such as hydromorphone.

B. Start a low-dose benzodiazepine.

C. Discontinue the morphine and focus on treatment with nonopioids.

D. Reassure Robert that this is a normal side effect and continue to increase the PCA for pain relief.

Correct Response and Analysis

Common side effects of opioids include constipation, myoclonus, nausea, somnolence, dry mouth, and pruritis. If bothersome to the patient, myoclonus can be addressed in a number of ways. A and B are the correct options. If the symptoms are distressing to the patient, a trial of opioid rotation or the addition of a benzodiazepine may be helpful.

C is incorrect; just because a patient has myoclonus with one opioid does not necessarily mean all other opioids will have the same effect.

D is incorrect because, although this is a known side effect, it is bothersome to the patient and increasing the morphine dose will likely worsen the myoclonus.

The Case Concludes

Robert's myoclonus resolves when the morphine is rotated to a hydromorphone PCA. He is tolerating palliative radiation and some limited physical therapy. A few days prior to discharge, you recommend a transition to oral pain medication. Robert is discharged on oxycodone extended release 60 mg every 12 hours based on his PCA requirements with oxycodone immediate release by mouth (PO) for breakthrough pain and dexamethasone PO. He has a follow-up appointment in the palliative care clinic and hematology/oncology clinic.

breathing. Concern also exists about respiratory depressant effects and the potential occurrence of opioid-induced hyperalgesia (OIH). Side effects are both dosage related and idiosyncratic; in the context of serious illness many adverse effects are determined by more than one factor. Whenever a side effect interferes with therapy, an assessment is needed to establish its etiologies and develop a responsive plan of care.

Constipation

Opioid-induced constipation is common and presumably worsened by advanced age, immobility, poor diet, intra-abdominal pathology, neuropathy, hypercalcemia, or the use of other constipating drugs.[105,106] Contributing causes should be minimized, if possible, and symptomatic therapies should be pursued. Prophylactic treatment at the time an opioid is prescribed is appropriate in those with predisposing factors; this is common in populations with serious or life-threatening illnesses.

Opioids produce constipation by slowing peristalsis and reducing GI secretion.[106] The opioid receptors that mediate these actions are both in the gut and CNS. All opioids can cause constipation, and this can occur when the drug is given by any route of administration. Considering the influence of receptors in the gut, it is likely that oral administration is more likely to produce constipation than drug delivery by other routes; the observation that transdermal fentanyl causes less constipation than oral morphine supports this conclusion.[70]

Diet changes (increased fiber and hydration) may be appropriate for patients with opioid-induced constipation. The consumption of more fiber should be considered only in those without debilitation or risk of bowel obstruction, which may increase the risk of bulk laxatives. During treatment, attention must be paid to privacy; a private commode with easy access is essential. Expense is another concern because the high cost of some laxatives can interfere with compliance.

Treatment

Few studies help define the comparative effectiveness of various constipation strategies and the potential value of dose escalation or combination therapy. Treatment usually begins with a simple oral regimen using a surfactant (eg, docusate) and an osmotic agent (eg, a poorly absorbed sugar such as lactulose, sorbitol, or polyethylene glycol) or a stimulant cathartic (eg, senna or bisacodyl). Dosages may be increased and the various agents may be administered in combination, as needed. **Table 17** provides an example of a stepwise laxative regimen.

Table 17. An Effective Stepwise Laxative Regimen

Step	Medication	Regimen
1	Docusate, 100 mg	1 cap twice daily
	Senna	1 tab twice daily
2	Increase senna	2 tabs twice daily
3	Increase senna	3 tabs twice daily
4	Increase senna	4 tabs twice daily
	and add	
	sorbitol	30 cc twice daily
	or	
	polyethylene glycol	17 g (1 tsp) in 8 oz of water daily
	or	
	bisacodyl	2 tabs twice daily
5	Increase sorbitol	30 cc three times daily
	or	
	polytheylene glycol	17 g in 8 oz of water twice daily
	or	
	bisacodyl	3 tabs three times daily

Refractory Constipation

Patients with refractory constipation may be considered for other therapies; most important among these is the peripherally acting opioid antagonist, methylnaltrexone.[105,107] This parenteral drug is efficacious in a majority of patients and usually produces a bowel movement within 1 hour; three doses (daily or every other day) may be needed to judge the maximal benefit of this drug. Adverse reactions include abdominal pain, usually described as "cramps" or "cramping," which generally are mild to moderate in severity, and decrease in incidence with subsequent dosing.[108] Other peripherally acting antagonists are in development, and oral naloxone may also be used.[105,107] Alvimopan, an oral agent, is approved for postoperative use in hospitalized patients via a limited-access program, but it has also been effective for patients with opioid-induced constipation.[109] Opioid antagonists should be considered only when the presence of mechanical obstruction has been excluded.

Severe Constipation

Rectal suppositories and enemas are rarely needed when a laxative regimen is conscientiously followed. These approaches may be appropriate if severe constipation develops, however. In this situation bowel obstruction should be ruled out and clearance of low impaction, if present, may be needed. Rectal bisacodyl (one to two suppositories) or high-volume enemas may be considered along with aggressive oral therapies such as sorbitol, lactulose, or polyethylene glycol, two to six times daily until a bowel movement occurs.

Nausea and Vomiting

When first prescribed, opioids may induce nausea and vomiting in 10% to 40% of patients.[110] Patients and families may be told that these problems are typically temporary and are not signs of an allergy. Opioids cause nausea through multiple mechanisms: activation of the chemoreceptor trigger zone in the fourth ventricle and the medullary vomiting center, stimulation of the vestibular system, and stimulation of the afferent cholinergic pathway from opioid-induced constipation.[110]

Symptomatic therapies, and, in some cases, opioid rotation, are the usual first steps in treatment. There is no proven benefit of one antiemetic medication over another, and there are no established guidelines for monotherapy, combination therapy, or dosing. Based on clinical experience, it may be valuable to query the patient about the extent to which nausea is movement-related or associated with vertiginous feelings, and the extent to which it follows the attempt to eat. Other questions relate to the link between specific medications, such as the opioid rescue dose, and worsening of the nausea and the connection between nausea and reflux symptoms or constipation. The responses to these questions may help rationalize therapy (see UNIPAC 4).

The nausea associated with an opioid may have other contributing factors and, if possible, disease-modifying therapies or reduction of other emetogenic treatments should be considered. Symptomatic therapy typically is added concurrently. Although first-line treatment for nausea believed to be opioid related usually is one of the dopamine blockers such as metaclopramide, prochlorperazine, haloperidol, or olanzepine or one of the 5-HT$_3$ antagonists such as ondansetron, cotherapy based on the symptom's characteristics may be justified. Movement-related nausea suggests prominent involvement of the vestibular-labyrinth system and suggests a trial of a drug used for vertigo, such as meclizine or scopolamine. Postprandial nausea suggests gastroparesis and may indicate first-line use of metaclopramide. Nausea associated with reflux symptoms suggests coadministration of a proton-pump inhibitor such as omeprazole, and nausea associated with fluctuating constipation should lead to more aggressive laxative therapy.

Nonpharmacologic treatments also should be considered. These may include acupuncture or acupressure, cognitive strategies, or dietary manipulation.

Somnolence, Mental Clouding, and Confusion

When opioid therapy is initiated, temporary sedation is common. This usually subsides within days unless concomitant disorders exist. Some patients initially are sleepy because sleep deprivation associated with pain is finally relieved. Some patients, however, experience long-lasting somnolence, mental clouding, or confusion, and some have other effects on higher cortical functioning such as mood disturbance (typically dysphoria) or perceptual disturbances. Frank delirium, in which any or all of these effects are combined with a fluctuating level of consciousness, may be caused or worsened by opioids and is common in the setting of far-advanced illness.

If somnolence or mental clouding occurs when opioid therapy has begun or when the dose is increased, this may signal poor opioid responsiveness and indicate the need for an alternative approach such as opioid rotation. When pain is relatively well controlled and opioid side effects are not severe, an alternative strategy is to treat somnolence through coadministration of a psychostimulant such as methylphenidate (5 mg once or twice per day to start, then titrated) or modafinil (100 mg to 200 mg in the morning to start, then increased once or twice).[111] These drugs can cause anxiety, tremulousness, insomnia, or anorexia, and all of these potential side effects must be monitored. Donepezil, a cholinesterase inhibitor, also has been reported to treat sedation; however, a trial may be limited by nausea.[112]

Patients who develop delirium should be evaluated for reversible factors. In the population with advanced illness, the etiologies are commonly multiple and the extent to which opioids contribute may be difficult to determine. To control the symptoms of delirium, the addition of a neuroleptic (such as haloperidol starting at a low dose, such as 0.5 mg orally or IV and titrating upwards) is appropriate even if the patient has the hypoactive type and seems outwardly calm. If agitation accompanies confusion, coadministration of a benzodiazepine along with the neuroleptic may be needed to achieve prompt behavioral control.

The atypical neuroleptics such as olanzepine or risperidone are also used commonly to manage a confusional state. Concern about excess mortality in elderly patients from these drugs is balanced by the lesser risk of extrapyramidal toxicity. These risks and benefits should be weighed when selecting a drug[113-116] (see *UNIPAC 4*).

Myoclonus

Myoclonus, or the sudden jerking movement of one or more muscles, is a sign of encephalopathy and may occur alone in the setting of opioid therapy or in association with somnolence or mental clouding. In populations with advanced illness, it is usually caused by some combination of factors. Patients and families may require reassurance about its meaning and treatment may or may not be necessary. If the movements are distressing and causative factors cannot be adequately eliminated, opioid rotation[117] or a trial of a benzodiazepine (usually clonazepam), an anticonvulsant (such as gabapentin), or baclofen can be considered.[118,119]

Respiratory Depression

The most serious potential toxicity associated with opioid drugs is respiratory depression. Opioids shift the CO_2-response curve and can lead to bradypnea followed by respiratory arrest. Unless there is acute massive overdose, this always occurs in association with somnolence. A drowsy patient with slowed breathing can be experiencing opioid overdose; an anxious patient with tachypnea is not manifesting primary opioid toxicity.

As long as opioid doses are incremented in safe steps as outlined above, respiratory depression is rare. Tolerance to the respiratory effects of opioid drugs develops quickly, but it is important to recognize that there may be loss of respiratory reserve in opioid-tolerant patients with normal respiratory rate and volume. This loss of reserve is reflected in persistence of the shift in CO_2 response. Clinically, it may contribute to the outcome when some other cardiopulmonary insult occurs. Opioid-treated patients who develop pneumonia or pulmonary embolism accompanied by respiratory compromise may demonstrate improved breathing if naloxone is given. This observation does not mean that the primary problem is opioid related; however, it suggests that a patient who suddenly develops respiratory depression while receiving a stable dose of an opioid should have other causes investigated even if naloxone reverses the problem.

Overdose

If opioid overdose is suspected and the patient is drowsy and breathing slowly, the opioid should be stopped and the patient can be monitored until the medication wears off; verbal or gentle mechanical stimulation may be needed to maintain arousal. Subsequently, the opioid can usually be restarted at a lower dose. On the rare occasion that naloxone is necessary, the best approach is to dilute 0.4 mg in 10 mL of saline and give 1 mL of this diluted mixture IV every 5 minutes until partial reversal occurs. Use of a dilute solution reduces the risk of a massive withdrawal response in physically dependent patients. Repeating the naloxone administration process or providing a naloxone infusion after initial dosing may be necessary because naloxone has a shorter half-life than most opioids.

Other Adverse Effects

The occurrence of dry mouth, sweating, or pruritis may present other targets for concurrent treatment. Among other less well-recognized effects, opioid-induced hypogonadism and sleep-disordered breathing are of greatest concern.

Opioid-Induced Hypogonadism

Opioid-induced hypogonadism is common[120] and raises concerns about the potential for sexual dysfunction, fatigue, accelerated bone loss, and mood disturbance. In medically ill patients, multiple contributing factors are likely, and there is little evidence to guide treatment. Among men with symptoms that may be related, measurement of testosterone and free testosterone should be considered if the goals of care would support a trial of testosterone-replacement therapy. In women there is more uncertainty about the role of hormone replacement, but in the appropriate context a patient with symptoms that could be related to hypogonadism should be considered for evaluation and treatment.

Sleep-Disordered Breathing

Sleep-disordered breathing is a poorly recognized adverse effect of opioid drugs.[121] Its prevalence and impact in medically ill populations are not known. In the appropriate setting, patients with symptoms (such as fatigue) that may be related to a sleep disorder and those with risk factors for sleep apnea syndrome (such as obesity or snoring) may warrant evaluation with a polysomnography.

Opioid-Induced Hyperalgesia

Opioid-induced hyperalgesia (OIH) is a physiological phenomenon that manifests in both in vitro and animal models, whereby opioid exposure lowers the threshold for response of nociceptive neurons and leads to hyperalgesic responses to noxious stimuli. Although its scientific demonstration has been invoked to explain the anecdotal occurrence of escalating pain in the absence of worsening pathology during opioid therapy,[122] the role of OIH in humans undergoing treatment for pain is not known.[123] Concern about OIH should not be used to justify withholding or limiting opioid therapy. Patients and families should not be told that opioids cause pain to worsen. At the same time, however, clinical observations suggest that OIH may be considered a rare cause of escalating pain if the pain occurs in the absence of clearly progressive pathology during aggressive opioid titration, and particularly if it is accompanied by tremulousness, confusion, or skin sensitivity. When suspected, it is reasonable to consider opioid rotation or the use of a nonopioid intervention for pain control to permit opioid dose reduction.

Opioid Risk Management

During the past 2 decades the substantial increase in prescription drug abuse and overdose deaths in the United States[124] has paralleled an increase in the use of opioid therapy for patients with chronic noncancer pain. These phenomena have raised substantial concerns on the part of the clinical community, regulators, policy makers, and those in law enforcement, and major changes in regulations governing prescribing are being implemented as a result.[54] Although clinicians must continue to advocate strongly for ready access to opioids for legitimate medical purposes, it is essential that they also acknowledge the serious nature of drug abuse and addiction, and the obligation to minimize these outcomes if possible.[125,126]

Risk assessment requires an understanding of key phenomena.[127] Addiction and physical dependence are different and should not be confused in the clinical setting; the capacity for withdrawal should never be stigmatized by the label of "addiction." *Pseudoaddiction* is a poorly characterized phenomenon and is best understood as the potential for unrelieved pain to drive aberrant behavior in some people. Importantly, pseudoaddiction and addiction can coexist, and the possibility of the former should not undermine the diagnosis of addiction or the appropriate management strategies to deal with seriously problematic drug-related behavior. Drug abuse refers to the use of any drug outside of social norms, and in the medical context also refers to egregious misuse of prescription drugs. Misuse and abuse of prescription drugs may also be characterized generically as aberrant drug-related behavior or nonadherence behavior[126] (see sidebar below for definitions of these terms).

Definitions[128]

Addiction.* *Addiction* is a primary, chronic, and neurobiologic disease. Its development and manifestations are influenced by genetic, psychosocial, and environmental factors. It is characterized by behaviors that include one or more of the following: impaired control over drug use, compulsive use, continued use despite harm, and craving.

Physical dependence.* *Physical dependence* is a state of adaptation indicated by a medication class-specific withdrawal syndrome that can be produced by abrupt cessation, rapid dosage reduction, decreasing blood level of the drug, or administration of an antagonist.

Pseudoaddiction. *Pseudoaddiction* is an iatrogenic syndrome with behaviors that mimic addiction and are driven by unrelieved pain. It is caused by inadequately prescribed analgesics, leading to patient demands for opioid analgesia that the care team considers excessive. When patients are provided with adequate dosages of medications at regular dosing intervals, the drug-seeking behaviors generally cease.

From Definitions related to the use of opioids for the treatment of pain by the American Pain Society, 2008, American Pain Society website, www.ampainsoc.org. © 2008 by American Pain Society. Reprinted with permission.

All prescribers, including those in the palliative care setting, should accept the need for universal risk management[129] during opioid therapy (**Table 18**). Managing the risks of abuse, addiction, and diversion can reduce both individual harm and potential harm to public health. The ability to manage risk also enhances expertise in prescribing to diverse populations, including those characterized by comorbid substance use disorder.

Clarifying Misconceptions About Opioids

Many physicians are reluctant to prescribe opioids because of misconceptions about their effects. Nurses may be reluctant to administer (and patients may be reluctant to use) morphine or other opioids for many of the same reasons. Similarly, patients and their family caregivers may have strong negative feelings about opioid analgesics. Healthcare professionals must be knowledgeable to avoid reinforcing fears and to dispel concerns that interfere with safe and effective prescribing. Some of these misconceptions were noted previously; the following and others are worthy of emphasis.

Opioids and Respiratory Depression

Clinically significant respiratory depression is extremely rare when patients receive appropriately titrated doses of an opioid. This is true of all patients, including those with serious cardiopulmonary disease. In fact, opioids have been shown to reduce the sensation of dyspnea without causing respiratory depression.[130]

When a terminally ill patient who has been receiving a stable dose of an opioid for several days or more develops signs of impending death, the appropriate action is to talk with the patient's family about the dying process, not to order naloxone. Symptoms and signs that signal imminent death include decreased or erratic respirations

in conjunction with extreme weakness; obtundation and confusion; and cool extremities. A few terminally ill patients die in a hyperventilatory state as a result of sepsis, acidosis, or respiratory muscle fatigue.

Opioids and Addiction

Addiction is a serious biopsychosocial disease with a strong genetic basis. Some patients with life-limiting illnesses will have this disease or the biological basis for it. The most accepted risk factors are a personal history of alcoholism or drug abuse, a family history of alcoholism or drug abuse, and major psychiatric disorder. The *de novo* development of addiction in a patient without any of these characteristics is distinctly rare. The need to prescribe opioids to patients who have a history of drug abuse or other predisposing factors to addiction is relatively common. As described previously, the most prudent course for prescribers is to adopt a universal precautions risk management strategy. This implies that all patients are appropriately assessed for risk and that actions commensurate with risk are taken to minimize the adverse outcomes of abuse, addiction, and diversion (Table 17). Clinicians cannot discount the importance of these latter outcomes; rather, they must recognize their characteristics, assess appropriately, and plan a management strategy to minimize risk at all times. Patients with a past history of an addiction disorder may be fearful of rekindling this disease. Special consideration and counseling need to be provided to these patients to optimize pain control and minimize psychological comorbidity.

In contrast to addiction, physical dependence is an expected result of long-term opioid treatment. It refers to the potential for withdrawal and is rarely a clinical problem as long as the dose is not abruptly lowered or an opioid antagonist is administered. Opioid withdrawal is characterized by the presence of one or more of a variable

Table 18. Principles of Risk Management During Opioid Therapy for Pain

Principle	Goals	Strategies	Comment
Stratify risk	Clarify the likelihood of future aberrant drug-related behavior.	Consider higher risk if • history of alcohol or drug abuse • family history of alcohol or drug abuse • major psychiatric disorder Other factors that suggest risk • cancer associated with heavy alcohol use or smoking • current heavy smoking • younger age • history of automobile accidents, chronic unemployment, limited support system Factors that may mitigate risk • poor performance status • limited prognosis • active recovery program	All patients should undergo risk assessment and stratification. Although many questionnaires have been developed to predict aberrant behavior or addiction, the clinical assessment is generally used in practice.
Structure therapy commensurate with risk	Develop practices to match monitoring with risk and, when needed, help patients maintain control	Strategies include • use of urine drug screening • small amounts prescribed • no use of short-acting drugs • use of one pharmacy • pill counts at time of visit • required consultations	The decision to implement one or more of these strategies is a matter of clinical judgment.
Assess drug-related behaviors over time	Track drug use in tandem with all relevant outcomes	Monitor drug-related behavior (eg, the need for early refills, obtaining multiple prescriptions, etc). Also monitor • pain relief • adverse drug effects • effect of drug on other outcomes	Broad monitoring of outcomes is consistent with integration of pain management into a palliative care model.
Respond to aberrant drug-related behaviors	Clinician compliance with laws and regulations Identifying patients needing additional management	If the patient engages in aberrant drug-related behavior, reassess and diagnose (addiction, other psychiatric disorder, pseudoaddiction, family issues, criminal intent) If diversion into the illicit market is occuring, prescribing should cease.	Even advanced illness does not free clinicians from complying with laws and regulations.

continued

Table 18. Principles of Risk Management During Opioid Therapy for Pain *continued*

Principle	Goals	Strategies	Comment
Document and communicate	Risk assessment and management should be viewed as integral to safe and effective prescribing.	Document • plan for monitoring and education of patients and families • monitoring of drug-related behavior on a regular basis • response if aberrant behavior occurs	It is valuable to openly discuss the need for universal risk management with other clinicians to reduce the risk of stigmatizing patients.

From Treatment of cancer pain, by RK Portenoy, 2011, Lancet, 377(9784), 2236-2247. © 2011 by Elsevier. Reprinted with permission.

group of symptoms and signs, including tremulousness, anxiety, insomnia, tachycardia, tachypnea, hypertension, nausea and vomiting, diarrhea, piloerection, and sweating. It is distinctly uncomfortable but not life threatening unless medical comorbidities increase the risk of tachycardia and hypertension. If a treatment, such as radiation therapy reduces the source of pain, an opioid can be tapered off without serious withdrawal symptoms in the vast majority of patients. Physical dependence should be anticipated and managed. It should never be confused with or labeled as addiction[128] or used to justify withholding of treatment.

Opioids and Tolerance

Tolerance is a state of adaptation through which exposure to a drug induces changes that result in the diminished effects of a drug over time. Tolerance to opioid-related adverse effects such as respiratory depression is a favorable phenomenon that greatly increases the safety of these drugs. Tolerance to analgesia, if it occurs, may be problematic, necessitating the use of higher doses that may preclude effective pain management. Some clinicians are so concerned about analgesic tolerance they advocate "saving" the drug until life expectancy is short. This is inappropriate. Clinically significant analgesic tolerance is an unusual problem in the clinical setting.

After an effective baseline dose is established, requirements usually plateau until the disease progresses, at which time the dosage is increased to control increased levels of pain. This course indicates that opioids should be used when pain severity warrants this therapy and that the therapy should never be delayed because of concern about loss of efficacy over time.

Opioids and Risk of Hastened Death

Clinicians may withhold opioid therapy to address ongoing pain because of concerns that the opioid drug will hasten death in patients with far-advanced illness who are likely to die in the near future. This is both a clinical and ethical challenge. Yes, opioid therapy can reduce respiratory reserve. Data from large observational studies are reassuring, however, and suggest that the influence of opioids on the timing of death is nil or minor in most cases.[131,132] Nevertheless, the possibility of hastening death or prolonging life cannot be entirely negated. Clinicians should have a solid understanding of the ethical basis for continuing effective opioid therapy in this context. Some clinicians refer to the ethical principle of double effect to provide a supportive framework and to help guide practice and educate others (see *UNIPAC 6*). Others rely solely on careful assessment of risks and benefits when recommending therapies intended for symptom relief and comfort in the terminal setting; these clinicians do not think that the principle of double effect is needed to justify treatment (see sidebar).

Principle of Double Effect

The principle of double effect notes that an action with known potential adverse consequences such as the administration of an opioid, may be undertaken when the following specific conditions apply[133]:

1. The action (such as giving opioids) must not be morally wrong.

2. The good effect (pain relief) must be the intended one.

3. The bad side effect (respiratory depression) cannot be the means by which the good effect is obtained.

4. The good effect must outweigh the bad side effect.

This principle has been used to justify the use of opioids to reduce pain and other forms of distress experienced by dying patients. With careful drug administration, the effective treatment of pain can proceed in a manner that is both relatively safe and informed by double effect.

Other Misconceptions

Lack of familiarity with long-term opioid therapy in medically ill populations may drive other misapprehensions that may be expressed by patients, family members, or professionals. Many people do not appreciate the extraordinary effective dose range of this drug class. Oral morphine, 2 mg every 4 hours may be an effective dose for some patients, while others may require the equivalent of grams per day. Repeated dose escalation in an effort to identify and retain a favorable balance between analgesia and side effects is appropriate; the occurrence of treatment-limiting side effects defines poor responsiveness to the regimen and requires a change in therapy.

Another misconception relates to routes of administration. Some perceive that parenteral drugs are more efficacious than oral drugs. With opioid compounds, efficacy is related to dose, and in most cases equivalent analgesia between the oral and parenteral routes is possible with dose adjustment. The decision to employ parenteral therapy requires other rationales such as the faster onset of effect from a bolus dose (eg, for the treatment of breakthrough pain), the possibility of more reliable absorption (eg, in patients with bowel pathology), or the need to lessen GI toxicity, which may be greater during oral treatment.

Some patients mistake itch and urticaria, known side effects of opioids, for signs of a true allergy. Others perceive nausea in this way. Although true hypersensitivity reactions can occur as the result of taking opioid drugs, they are distinctly rare and, in most cases, patients can be given the drug with cotherapy to reduce the side effect.

Nonopioid Analgesics

Acetaminophen (also known as paracetamol) and NSAIDs comprise the nonopioid analgesics available in the United States. The analgesic mechanism of acetaminophen is poorly understood but may involve inhibition of prostaglandin formation in the CNS. In contrast to NSAIDs, acetaminophen is not anti-inflammatory. Given its favorable safety profile, it may be considered for the long-term treatment of mild pain, notwithstanding scant evidence that the combination of acetaminophen plus an opioid is more efficacious than an opioid alone.[134-137]

Acetaminophen

Acetaminophen has a narrow therapeutic window. In the United States, concerns about unintentional overdose have been rising, and regulators are now limiting the amount of acetaminophen to 325 mg/dose, suggesting that a maximum dose should be 2.6 g/day (eight tablets per day of a formulation containing 325 mg per dose unit[138]). Regulators suggest that patients with significant liver disease or heavy alcohol use should be considered to have a relative contraindication to this drug.

Nonsteroidal Anti-Inflammatory Drugs

NSAIDs are diverse drugs (**Table 19**)[139] that produce analgesia by inhibiting the enzyme cyclo-oxygenase (COX) in the periphery and CNS, thereby reducing tissue levels of peripheral and central prostaglandins. There are two main forms of COX: a form that largely is constitutive (COX-1) and a form that largely is induced during the inflammatory cascade (COX-2). All NSAIDs inhibit both COX-1 and COX-2, but with varying selectivity.

NSAIDs have analgesic, anti-inflammatory, and antipyretic effects. They are effective analgesics in combination with opioids[140,141] and may be especially useful in patients with bone pain or pain that is related to gross inflammatory lesions. They appear to be less useful in patients who have neuropathic pain.

A risk assessment will strongly influence the selection of patients with serious illness for a trial of NSAID therapy. The patient risk profile assessment is an essential step in the decision to try or withhold NSAID therapy.

All NSAIDs produce GI toxicity, which ranges from pain, nausea, or heartburn to ulceration and bleeding. Drugs that are more selective for COX-2 are relatively less likely to produce side effects related to COX-1 inhibition, such as GI toxicity. Drugs specifically developed as selective COX-2 inhibitors have been shown to produce fewer GI effects when low-dose aspirin therapy is not taken concurrently.[142] Limited data suggest that some of the nonselective NSAIDs (ibuprofen, naproxen, nabumetone, and the nonacetylated salicylates such as choline magnesium trisalicylate and salsalate) also pose a relatively lower risk for this toxicity.[143,144] Regardless of the drug, the risk of serious GI toxicity is higher in those older than 60 years, those with a history of an ulcer or GI hemorrhage, those receiving a corticosteroid or anticoagulant, and those receiving a high dose of the NSAID. *H. pylori* also may be a risk factor, and patients with a history of gastritis or ulcer disease can be tested for this infection. NSAIDs should be considered relatively contraindicated in patients with multiple risk factors. Those with only one or two risk factors should be strongly considered for treatment with a selective COX-2 inhibitor (celecoxib) or a coadministered gastroprotective drug, usually a proton-pump inhibitor.[145]

All NSAIDs also produce cardiovascular toxicities, which include fluid retention (associated with blood pressure elevation and risk of volume overload) and prothrombotic effects. The prothrombotic effect, which appears to be related to inhibition of the COX-2 enzyme, predisposes to angina and myocardial infarction, transient ischemic attack and stroke, and symptomatic peripheral vascular disease.[142] Mostly as a result of the latter concern, two COX-2 selective NSAIDs were taken off the US market and others have not been approved. Subsequent research has concluded that cardiovascular toxicity characterizes all NSAIDs, and there is large drug-related variation in this risk.[146] Indeed, the only labeled COX-2 selective drug in the United States at press time, celecoxib, appears to pose a far lower risk than other drugs in this class; similarly, some of the nonselective drugs such as naproxen and ibuprofen appear to present relatively lower risk for these cardiovascular events.

With the exception of the nonacetylated salicylates (choline magnesium trisalicylate and salsalate) and the selective COX-2 inhibitors (celecoxib), all NSAIDs interfere with platelet aggregation. Despite its short half-life, aspirin irreversibly inhibits platelet aggregation for the lifetime of the platelet (4-7 days); the inhibitory effect of other NSAIDs lasts about 2 days. NSAID

Table 19. NSAIDs and Related Analgesics[139]

GENERIC NAME	APPROXIMATE HALF-LIFE (HOURS)	STARTING DAILY DOSAGE	MAXIMUM DAILY DOSAGE	EXCRETION	COMMENTS*
Para-Aminophenol Derivatives					
Acetaminophen	2-4	650 mg-1,000 mg every 4-6 hours	4,000 mg	85% renal	Lacks peripheral anti-inflammatory and antiplatelet effect. Excessive dosing leads to liver toxicity. Monitor platelet and liver function with chronic disease.
Nonsteroidal Anti-Inflammatory Analgesics					
Salicylates					
Acetylsalicylic acid (aspirin)	3-12	325 mg-650 mg every 4 hours	6,000 mg	100% renal	May inhibit platelet aggregation for > 1 week. Contraindicated for children with fever or other viral syndromes.
Choline magnesium trisalicylate	8-12	Initial dose: 1,500 mg, then 1,500 mg every 8-12 hours; 750 mg every 8-12 hours for elderly patients	4,500 mg	100% renal	Approved for children Minimal GI toxicity Suspension available Minimal platelet effects
Diflunisal	8-12	Initial dose: 1,000 mg, then 500 mg every 12 hours	1,500 mg	90% renal, < 5% fecal	N/A
Salsalate	8-12	Initial dose: 1,500 mg, then 1,500 mg every 12 hours	3,000 mg	100% renal	Minimal platelet effects
Propionic Acids					
Flurbiprofen	5-6	50 mg-100 mg every 6-8 hours	300 mg	65%-85% renal	N/A
Ibuprofen	2-4	400 mg-600 mg every 6-8 hours	3,200 mg	50%-75% renal	Suspension formulation available
Ketoprofen	2-4	75 mg every 8 hours or 50 mg every 6 hours; 25-50 mg every 8 hours for mild renal impairment and elderly patients	300 mg	50%-90% renal, 1%-8% fecal	N/A
Naproxen	13	Initial dose: 500 mg, then 250 mg every 6-8 hours	1,500 mg	95% renal	Cautious use of > 1,500 mg/day may be more efficacious. Suspension available.
Oxaprozin	50-60; 40 with repeated dosing	1,200 mg daily	1,800 mg	60% renal, 30%-35% fecal	N/A

continued

Table 19. NSAIDs and Related Analgesics[139] *continued*

GENERIC NAME	APPROXIMATE HALF-LIFE (HOURS)	STARTING DAILY DOSAGE	MAXIMUM DAILY DOSAGE	EXCRETION	COMMENTS*
Nonsteroidal Anti-Inflammatory Analgesics *cont.*					
Acetic Acids					
Diclofenac	2	50 mg every 8-12 hours	150 mg	50%-70% renal, 30%-35% fecal	A 1% topical gel is available for osteoarthritis.
Indomethacin	4-5	25 mg-50 mg every 8-12 hours	200 mg	60% renal, 30% fecal	Available in sustained release and rectal formulations. Greater GI and CNS toxicity. Not recommended for elderly patients.
Sulindac	8-16	150 mg every 12 hours	400 mg	50% renal, 25% fecal	N/A
Tolmetin	1	400 mg every 8 hours	1,800 mg	100% renal	N/A
Oxicam					
Piroxicam	50	20 mg daily	20 mg	67% renal, 33% fecal	Progressive increase in response may occur because of long half-life; steady state 7-12 days after initiation of therapy
Fenamates					
Meclofenamic acid	50 minutes to 3.3 hours	50 mg-100 mg every 4-6 hours	400 mg	67% renal, 20%-25% fecal	Dose-related diarrhea
Mefenamic acid	2	Loading dose: 500 mg; then 250 mg every 6 hours	1,000 mg	67% renal, 33% fecal	Intended for short-term use; dose-related diarrhea
COX-2 Inhibitors					
Celecoxib	11	100 mg twice daily; can give 400 mg on first day of administration	200 mg after first day of administration	97% hepatic metabolism, 3% renal	Less GI toxicity

Increased cardiovascular events

Minimal platelet effects |
| **Pyrrolopyrrole** | | | | | |
| Ketorolac | 4-6 | IV/IM: 30 mg every 6 hours; 15 mg every 6 hours for elderly patients.

PO: 10 mg every 4-6 hours | IV/IM: 120 mg; 60 mg for elderly patients

PO: 40 mg | 91% renal, 6% fecal | Usually used as single dose IV/IM. Maximum duration is 5 days. |

continued

Table 19. NSAIDs and Related Analgesics[139] *continued*

GENERIC NAME	APPROXIMATE HALF-LIFE (HOURS)	STARTING DAILY DOSAGE	MAXIMUM DAILY DOSAGE	EXCRETION	COMMENTS*
Pyranocarboxylic Acids					
Etodolac	6-7	200 mg-400 mg every 6-8 hours	1,200 mg	60% renal, 27% fecal	N/A
Naphthlalkanones					
Nabumetone	23-30	1,000 mg	2,000 mg	Renal	N/A

BUN, blood urea nitrogen; CNS, central nervous system; CV, cardiovascular; GI, gastrointestinal; IM, intramuscular; IV, intravenous; PO, by mouth.

* Use the lowest effective dosage for the shortest possible duration; see warnings below and as published for each drug.

Starting and maximal dosages are not intended to preclude clinical judgment of the prescriber. A dosage reduction is recommended for elderly patients, those with renal insufficiency, and when multiple medications are taken. Dosages can be incremented weekly. Studies of NSAIDs in the cancer population are limited. Dosing guidelines are based on studies in inflammatory diseases; consequently, dosages in patients with cancer are empiric.

NSAIDs can cause severe or life-threatening CV, GI, and renal toxicities, especially in elderly and chronically ill patients or if prescribed at high dosages over longer periods. If they must be used under high-risk circumstances, consider regular monitoring of stools for occult blood and BUN, creatinine, and liver function.

therapy generally is avoided in patients with a bleeding diathesis of any type.

All NSAIDS can adversely affect renal function. The range of potential lesions is large and includes acute interstitial nephritis, acute tubular necrosis in patients with low renal perfusion, and chronic nephropathy. NSAIDs also should be avoided in patients who are dehydrated, have renal insufficiency, or who have disorders associated with a high likelihood of renal dysfunction (eg, multiple myeloma).

Significant hepatotoxicity from NSAID therapy is uncommon, but mild elevations in liver enzymes are frequently encountered. In the context of serious illness, stable and mild elevations should be monitored over time and the drug may be continued if it is providing benefit.

Considering this range of toxicities, the decision to offer a trial of NSAID treatment should take into account the likelihood of benefit and the risk of adverse effects, as well as the cost and burden associated with prolonged treatment. Risk profiling should inform drug selection, which in most cases would begin with one of the drugs known to pose a relatively lower risk for GI toxicity (eg, celecoxib) or a drug with relatively low cardiovascular toxicity (naproxen).[144,146] Regardless of the drug selected, lower doses are associated with less risk than higher doses. Most patients have one or more risk factors for GI toxicity, so concurrent use of a gastroprotective drug such as omeprazole also can be considered.

Because there is substantial variability in patient response to the various NSAIDs, the decision to try an NSAID may require several trials to identify the agent with the most favorable risk-to-benefit ratio. Past response to a NSAID may inform current drug selection, and pharmacokinetic considerations (eg, use of a drug with once-daily or twice-daily administration) also may be important.

Adjuvant Analgesics

The term *adjuvant analgesic* originally was coined to refer to a small number of drugs that were marketed for indications other than pain but were found to be potentially useful as analgesics in patients receiving opioid therapy. During the past 3 decades, the number, diversity, and uses of these drugs have increased dramatically, and several now are indicated as first-line therapy for certain types of pain.[147] As a result, the term, adjuvant analgesic, has become somewhat of a misnomer, but it still is commonly applied in the context of cancer pain. The term is used interchangeably with coanalgesic.

Adjuvant analgesics often are considered for treatment of chronic pain when a patient is poorly responsive to opioids (ie, inability to titrate the opioid to a dose that maintains a favorable balance between analgesia and side effects). The addition of an adjuvant analgesic is one approach among many that may be considered for such patients.[148] With the exception of certain pain states for which specific drugs have been identified as potential first-line therapies, a trial of a coanalgesic usually should be considered only after efforts have been made to optimize opioid therapy.

The large and growing number of adjuvant analgesics (**Table 20**) can be categorized on the basis of how they are used in clinical practice.[147] Based upon conventional practice, the categories of available agents include
- drugs potentially useful for any type of pain (multipurpose analgesics)
- drugs used to treat neuropathic pain
- drugs used for bone pain
- drugs used for pain and other symptoms in the setting of bowel obstruction
- drugs specifically formulated for primary headache disorders.

Multipurpose Analgesics

Some drug classes have been studied in diverse types of chronic pain, including corticosteroids, antidepressants, alpha-2 adrenergic agonists, cannabinoids, and topical therapies. These drugs have broad indications.

Glucocorticoids

In palliative care, corticosteroids are used to address pain, nausea, fatigue, anorexia, and malaise.[149-151] Based on extensive observations, these drugs may be analgesic for neuropathic and bone pain, pain associated with capsular expansion or duct obstruction, pain from bowel obstruction, pain caused by lymphedema, and headache caused by increased intracranial pressure. The mechanism of analgesia probably relates to reduction of tumor-related edema, antiinflammatory effects, and direct effects on pain pathways.

Dexamethasone is usually preferred, presumably because of its long half-life and relatively low mineralocorticoid effects. There is no evidence, however, that this drug is safer or more effective than other corticosteroids. A typical regimen is 1 mg to 2 mg of dexamethasone orally or parenterally once or twice daily; this may be preceded by a larger loading dose of 10 mg to 20 mg. This regimen, or comparable regimens of alternative steroids, is based on clinical experience. Patients may do well with lower or higher doses or with once-daily rather than twice-daily dosing. Very high dose therapy (eg, dexamethasone, 50 mg to 100 mg IV), followed by 12 mg to 24 mg four times daily, tapered over 1 to 3 weeks, has been used empirically for pain crises related to bone or nerve injury. This approach was developed for treatment of emerging spinal cord compression and has been observed to yield rapid pain relief with acceptable risk of adverse effects.[152]

Long-term corticosteroid therapy may produce myopathy, worsening immunocompromise, psychotomimetic effects, and hypoadrenalism. These risks must be balanced against the observed benefit.

Analgesic Antidepressants

Antidepressants have been widely studied as analgesics for varied types of chronic pain.[147,153-156]

Table 20. Adjuvant Analgesics

DRUG CLASS	SUBCLASS	EXAMPLES	COMMENTS
Multipurpose Analgesics			
Glucocorticoids	N/A	Dexamethasone, prednisone	Used for bone pain, neuropathic pain, lymphedema pain, headache, bowel obstruction
Antidepressants	Tricyclics	Desipramine, amitriptyline	Used for opioid-refractory neuropathic pain first if comorbid depression; secondary amine compounds (eg, desipramine) have fewer side effects and may be preferred
	SNRIs	Duloxetine, milnacipran	Good evidence in some conditions but overall less than tricyclics; however, better side-effect profile; often tried first
	SSRIs	Paroxetine, citalopram	Very limited evidence, and if pain is the target, other subclasses preferred
	Other	Bupropion	Limited evidence but less sedating, and often tried early when fatigue or somnolence is a problem
Alpha-2 adrenergic agonists	N/A	Tizanidine, clonidine	Seldom used systemically because of side effects, but tizanidine is preferred for a trial; clonidine is used in neuraxial analgesia
Cannabinoid	N/A	THC/cannabidiol, nabilone, THC	Good evidence in cancer pain for THC/cannabidiol; limited evidence for other commercially available compounds
Topical agents	Anesthetic	Lidocaine patch Local anesthetic creams	N/A
	Capsaicin	8% patch; 0.25%, 0.75% creams	High-concentration patch indicated for postherpetic neuralgia
	NSAIDs	Diclofenac and others	Evidence in focal musculoskeletal pains
	Tricyclics	Doxepin cream	Used in itch; may be tried for pain
	Other		Compounded creams with varied drugs tried empirically, but no evidence
Used for Neuropathic Pain			
Multipurpose drugs	As above	As above	As above
Anticonvulsants	Gaba-pentinoids	Gabapentin, pregabalin	Used first for opioid-refractory neuropathic pain unless comorbid depression; may be multipurpose considering evidence in postsurgical pain; both drugs act at the N-type calcium channel in the CNS, but response to one or the other varies
	Other	Oxcarbazepine, lamotrigine, topiramate, lacosamide, divalproex, carbamazepine, phenytoin	Limited evidence for all examples listed; newer drugs preferred because of less side-effect liability, but individual variation is wide; all are considered for opioid-refractory neuropathic pain if antidepressants and gabapentinoids are ineffective
Sodium channel drugs	Sodium channel blockers	Mexiletine IV lidocaine	Good evidence for IV lidocaine

continued

Table 20. Adjuvant Analgesics *continued*

DRUG CLASS	SUBCLASS	EXAMPLES	COMMENTS
Sodium channel drugs (cont.)	Sodium channel modulator	Lacosamide	New anticonvulsant with limited evidence of analgesic effects
GABA agonists	GABA$_A$ agonist	Clonazepam	Limited evidence, but used for neuropathic pain with anxiety
	GABA$_B$ agonist	Baclofen	Evidence in trigeminal neuralgia is the basis for trials in other types of neuropathic pain.
N-methyl-D-aspartate inhibitors	N/A	Ketamine, memantine, others	Limited evidence for ketamine, but positive experience for IV use in advanced illness or a pain crisis; little evidence for oral drugs
Used for Bone Pain			
Bisphosphonates	N/A	Pamidronate, ibandronate, clodronate	Good evidence; like the NSAIDs or glucocorticoids, usually considered first-line therapy; also reduces other adverse skeletal-related events; concern about osteonecrosis of the jaw and renal insufficiency; may limit use
Calcitonin	N/A	N/A	Limited evidence but usually well tolerated
Radiopharma-ceuticals	N/A	Strontium-89, samarium-153	Good evidence, but limited use because of bone marrow effects and need for expertise
Used for Bowel Obstruction			
Anticholinergic drugs	N/A	Scopolamine (hyoscine) compounds, glycopyrrolate	Along with a glucocorticoid, considered first-line adjuvant for nonsurgical bowel obstruction
Somatostatin analogue	N/A	Octreotide	Along with a glucocorticoid, considered first-line adjuvant for nonsurgical bowel obstruction

CNS, central nervous system; GABA, gamma-aminobutyric acid; IV, intravenous; NSAID, nonsteroidal anti-inflammatory drug; SNRI, serotonin norepinephrine reuptake inhibitor; SSRI, selective serotonin reuptake inhibitor; THC, tetrahydrocannabinol.

From Treatment of cancer pain, by RK Portenoy, 2011, Lancet, 377(9784), 2236-2247. © 2011 by Elsevier. Reprinted with permission.

Although very few of these studies have included medically ill patients, the utility of these drugs in these populations is accepted. In opioid-treated populations with advanced medical illness, these drugs usually are considered for patients with refractory neuropathic pain.

Antidepressants produce analgesia independently of mood effects. Pain reduction may be enhanced, however, if there is a concurrent positive mood effect. The analgesic mode of action is thought to be related to enhanced availability of monoamines in descending pain-modulating systems. Inhibition of norepinephrine reuptake appears to be the most important mode of action, but serotonergic and dopaminergic effects probably play a role in analgesia.

The analgesic antidepressants may be categorized by subclasses. Analgesic efficacy is best established for some of the tricyclic compounds[153,157-159] and the serotonin-norepinephrine reuptake inhibitors (SNRIs)[156,159-162]; there is minimal evidence of analgesic efficacy with the serotonin selective reuptake inhibitors (SSRIs).[153,163,164] Limited evidence supports benefit from bupropion, a dopamine reuptake inhibitor.[165]

The tricyclic antidepressants include tertiary amines such as amitriptyline, and secondary amines such as nortriptyline and desipramine.

The secondary amines are more selective at noradrenergic reuptake sites, and they have a more favorable side-effect profile than amitriptyline. All tricyclic compounds are relatively contraindicated in patients with serious heart disease, severe prostatic hypertrophy, and narrow-angle glaucoma.

There is strong evidence that duloxetine, an SNRI, is analgesic.[161,162] There is less evidence for others in this class, including milnacipran, venlafaxine, and desvenlafaxine. The side effect profile of this class, which includes nausea, sexual dysfunction, and somnolence or mental clouding, usually is more favorable than even the secondary amine tricyclic drugs, but there is a great deal of individual variation. Among patients with serious medical illness, the first-line analgesic antidepressants may be either one of the secondary amine tricyclic compounds (usually desipramine) or duloxetine, and the decision between these drugs usually is based on a case-by-case assessment of risk and cost.

Other antidepressants usually are considered only if the drugs mentioned before are ineffective. The exception is bupropion, which is a dopamine and norepinephrine reuptake inhibitor that is distinguished by the tendency to be activating. A trial of bupropion sometimes is considered early on if pain is complicated by fatigue or somnolence, even though the evidence of analgesic efficacy is weak.

All of the analgesic antidepressants should be started at a relatively low initial dose. The starting dose for desipramine, for example, is 10 mg to 25 mg at night. The dose should be increased slowly until pain lessens or side effects occur. If analgesia is going to occur at any given dose, it usually appears within 1 week—much more quickly than antidepressant effects typically evolve. The usual effective dose of desipramine is between 50 mg and 150 mg per day, but if neither analgesia nor intolerable side effects occur, continued dose escalation is reasonable. Other antidepressants such as duloxetine or bupropion should similarly be started at a relatively low initial dose and titrated to conventional maximal doses to determine whether an analgesic or positive mood effect occurs.

In clinical practice lower doses of the tricyclic drugs are used for pain and sleep, (eg, desipramine 25 mg to 75 mg at bedtime). At relatively high doses of a tricyclic drug (above 100 mg per day) the plasma drug concentration and an electrocardigram should be checked. Tricyclic antidepressants can prolong the QTc interval and predispose to cardiac arrhythmias. These drugs should be used cautiously when a patient has known heart disease or is receiving other drugs that can prolong the QT interval, such as methadone.

Alpha-2 Adrenergic Agonists

Clonidine, which can be administered orally, transdermally, or intraspinally, has been studied in patients with chronic noncancer pain and was shown to be analgesic for both neuropathic and nociceptive pain in a controlled cancer pain trial.[166] There is less evidence of analgesic efficacy with oral tizanidine[167] and parenteral dexmedetomidine.[168] These drugs can produce somnolence and dry mouth and may cause hypotension. Considering these side effects and limited evidence of benefit, they are seldom used systemically for pain in medically ill populations. For those with refractory neuropathic pain or muscle spasm, tizanidine (which has less hypotensive effect than clonidine) may be considered for a cautious trial. Dosing may be initiated at bedtime to provide hypnotic effects.

Cannabinoids

Cannabinoids are derived from *cannabis* (marijuana) plants. They interact with an endogenous system that includes cannabinoid-like ligands (the endocannabinoids) and multiple receptors in both the periphery and CNS. Although concern about the abuse potential of cannabinoid drugs has slowed their development, several cannabinoid-type drugs are commercially available and others are under study. Data suggest that these compounds may be useful as multipurpose analgesics.[169-171] Nabiximols, an oromucosal spray that contains tetrahydrocannabinol plus cannabidiol (and smaller concentrations of other compounds), is approved in Canada and elsewhere (but not yet in the United States) for the treatment of spasticity and pain in multiple sclerosis and as an adjunctive treatment for pain in patients with advanced cancer.[172,173] Commercially available cannabinoids, specifically tetrahydrocannabinol and nabilone, may have analgesic effects but are rarely used for pain because of side effect liability. Until newer cannabinoid preparations become available in the United States, clinical use of cannabinoids for pain will likely be limited.

Topical Therapies
The most widely used topical therapies for pain contain local anesthetics. Lidocaine 5% patches[174] and various anesthetic gels or creams[175,176] may be applied to focal areas of pain related to nerve injury[177] or joint or soft tissue injury,[178] with the intent of producing analgesia. For the lidocaine patch, limited data indicate a high level of safety with four patches applied 24 hours a day for up to 72 hours.[179] Long-term therapy with this number of patches or fewer may be considered.

Capsaicin, a naturally occurring compound in chili pepper, depletes substance P from the terminals of afferent C-fibers. Topical application of a low-concentration cream (0.1%) potentially can benefit patients with various types of neuropathic and joint pain.[180] Burning, which usually is transitory, is the major side effect. Application three to four times daily for a period of at least 1 week is needed to determine benefit. In 2009 the US Food and Drug Administration approved a high-concentration capsaicin patch (8%) for treatment of postherpetic neuralgia.[181] This patch is applied for 1 hour in a monitored environment, and, if effective, can yield benefit for months.

Numerous anti-inflammatory drugs have been investigated for topical use, and at present a diclofenac patch, cream, and gel are commercially available in the United States. Although studied in musculoskeletal pain,[182] there is favorable anecdotal experience in diverse types of pain.

Topical tricyclic antidepressants may be analgesic[183] and a doxepin cream is commercially available. Doxepin cream is indicated for pruritus and may be considered for patients with local or regional pain, especially neuropathic painful itch.

Other drugs may be compounded into creams for patients with pain. The most popular are ketamine and gabapentin, but a variety of others are in use, including topical opioids. Supporting data for these therapies are meager or absent, but they appear to be safe. In the setting of refractory pain, a trial may be reasonable if cost is not prohibitive.

Drugs Used for Neuropathic Pain
All of the multipurpose analgesics are used for opioid-refractory neuropathic pain in medically ill people.[55] The analgesic antidepressants are widely considered to be first-line for this indication if pain is accompanied by depressed mood.[184] Other first-line drugs for neuropathic pain are anticonvulsants, specifically the gabapentinoids.

Anticonvulsants
Analgesic effects are best characterized for the gabapentinoids, gabapentin, and pregabalin. These drugs have been extensively studied in diverse types of neuropathic pain,[185-191] including fibromyalgia[192] and cancer-related neuropathic pain.[186] The analgesic mechanism for the gabapentinoids involves binding to the alpha-2 delta protein modulator of the N-type, voltage-gated

calcium channel, which reduces calcium influx into the neuron. The main difference between these drugs is pharmacokinetic. In contrast to pregabalin, gabapentin transit from gut to receptor depends on a saturable transporter in the small bowel and CNS. At a relatively high gabapentin dose (approximately 1,800 mg per day, but the dose can be higher or lower in individual cases), kinetics become nonlinear. Dosing of pregabalin is simpler, usually requires fewer steps to reach an effective dose range, and is not complicated by the potential for a kinetic plateau.

Neither gabapentin nor pregabalin are metabolized in the liver; renal excretion requires dose reduction in the setting of renal impairment. These drugs have no known drug-drug interactions. Their main side effects are mental clouding, dizziness, and somnolence; edema and weight gain are less common. Occasionally, lower-extremity edema progressing to heart failure can occur, which will warrant discontinuing the drug.

Gabapentin is often initiated at a dose of approximately 100 mg to 300 mg per day for medically frail patients. The dose is gradually titrated in two or three divided doses while monitoring analgesia and side effects. Dose escalation should extend to 3,600 mg per day, and, in the absence of a demonstrated analgesic ceiling or side effects, even higher doses may be tried. The starting dose of pregabalin is usually 50 mg to 75 mg per day, and escalation to the usual effective dose of 150 mg to 300 mg twice daily typically is accomplished in two to three steps over 1 week. The evidence shows that patients who are "gabapentin failures" may respond to pregabalin[193] and anecdotal observations exist; consequently, it is appropriate to consider a trial of pregabalin if an attempt with the first drug does not yield benefit.

Other Anticonvulsants

Many other anticonvulsants have been studied as analgesics and may be considered for trials if opioid-refractory neuropathic pain does not respond to gabapentinoids or analgesic antidepressants.[194] Older drugs such as carbamazepine,[195] valproate, and phenytoin have analgesic effects but a relatively higher adverse effect liability than newer agents. Among the new drugs, lamotrigine has been efficacious in several, but not all, studies of neuropathic pain,[196] but carries a small risk for serious cutaneous hypersensitivity and slow titration is required to reduce this risk. Oxcarbazepine, a metabolite of carbamazepine, has a safer pharmacologic profile and limited evidence of analgesic efficacy,[197] and there is equivocal support for topiramate.[198] Lacosamide, a sodium channel modulator, also yielded analgesic effects in one trial and may be considered if other drugs are not effective.[199] Finally, clonazepam, a benzodiazepine, is favored by some clinicians despite limited supporting data, presumably because its anxiolytic effects are positive.[200]

Other Drugs Used for Neuropathic Pain

Systemic sodium channel blockers, including IV lidocaine and oral antiarrhythmic drugs such as mexiletine, are analgesic.[201,202] A brief IV infusion of lidocaine, typically 2 mg/kg to 4 mg/kg infused over 20 to 30 minutes in a monitored setting, can be useful when prompt relief is needed for neuropathic pain and an opioid is not adequate. Oral mexiletine is rarely tried but is an option for refractory pain.[203]

There is some evidence that one of the commercially available NMDA receptor antagonists, ketamine, has analgesic properties.[204] Ketamine, a dissociative anesthetic, can provide analgesia when infused IV or SC at subanesthetic doses (eg, 0.1 mg/kg to 1.5 mg/kg per hour) or administered orally.[205] The side effect profile, which includes psychotomimetic effects and delirium, may be problematic, however, and the most common use is for short-term therapy in a monitored setting or for refactory terminal pain. Oral NMDA receptor antagonists such as memantine, amantadine, and dextromethorphan have less evidence in support of analgesic effects in neuropathic pain[206] and rarely are considered.

Drugs that interact directly with the gamma-aminobutyric acid (GABA) receptors comprise the GABA$_A$ antagonists, specifically the benzodiazepines, and the GABA$_B$ antagonists, which include baclofen. As noted before, the only benzodiazepine generally used for neuropathic pain is clonazepam. Baclofen, an antispasticity drug, has established efficacy in trigeminal neuralgia and is effective anecdotally for neuropathic pain of other types, including cancer pain.[207] A low starting dose of 5 mg twice daily can be gradually escalated to doses that may exceed 200 mg per day for some patients.

Drugs Used for Bone Pain

Patients with cancer who have multifocal bone pain are usually given an opioid combined with an NSAID or an adjuvant analgesic used specifically for bone pain. In addition to a corticosteroid such as dexamethasone, the adjuvant analgesics used in this setting include osteoclast inhibitors (bisphosphonates or calcitonin) and bone-seeking radionuclides.

Osteoclast Inhibitors

Bisphosphonates prevent skeletal-related events, including fracture, and substantial data support their analgesic potential.[11,208] This applies to all of the parenteral bisphosphonates including pamidronate, zoledronic acid, ibandronate, and clodronate (not available in the United States), as well as oral ibandronate and clodronate. A drug typically is chosen on the basis of experience, cost, and convenience.

The bisphosphonates generally are well tolerated. A transitory flu-like illness with a pain flare may be reported. The risk of nephrotoxicity, which usually is temporary, necessitates a check of renal function before treatment; if impaired, the starting dose should be lowered and the patient carefully monitored. Although bisphosphonate drugs are used to treat hypercalcemia, the development of symptomatic hypocalcemia following treatment is uncommon in normocalcemic patients who receive the drug for pain. Nonetheless, calcium levels should be monitored during therapy.

There are two other unusual but serious complications associated with the bisphonates: osteonecrosis of the jaw[209] and femur fracture.[210] These complications usually occur after months of treatment. Because oral trauma and dental infections increase risk for jaw osteonecrosis, patients with poor dentition should be considered to have a relative contraindication to this therapy.[211]

Calcitonin is another osteoclast inhibitor with potential analgesic effects in bone pain. Small controlled trials have yielded conflicting results,[212] however, and this drug usually is considered only if a bisphosphonate cannot be given.

Bone-Seeking Radionuclides

Bone-seeking radionuclides such as strontium-89 and samarium-153 link a short-lived radiation source to a bisphosphonate molecule. These compounds can be a useful treatment for multifocal bone pain.[213] There is evidence that they may provide complete pain relief in 1 to 6 months, but there is no evidence that one isotope or dose is superior to another.[214] Myelosuppression is the most significant concern and treatment requires special skills and facilities. If available, treatment with a bone-seeking radionuclide typically is considered for patients with refractory multifocal bone pain whose blood counts are not very low and who are not expected to require myelosuppressive chemotherapy in the near future.

Drugs Used for the Pain of Bowel Obstruction

Patients with advanced intra-abdominal or pelvic tumors may develop inoperable bowel obstruction associated with pain and other symptoms (see *UNIPAC 4*). Patients whose conditions cannot be managed by stenting[215] or tube decompression potentially can experience good symptom control with medical management.[216] The approach relies on hydration and opioid therapy combined with adjuvant analgesics that address pain, intraluminal secretions, and peristalsis. The latter drugs may include a corticosteroid,[217,218] anticholinergic drugs such as scopolamine or glycopyrrolate, and octreotide.

Anticholinergic Drugs

Scopolamine can be administered via a transdermal system or parenteral infusion. In the United States only the hydrobromide salt is available, which crosses the blood-brain barrier and may produce somnolence and confusion. *Glycopyrrolate* is an anticholinergic drug that has limited ability to cross the blood-brain barrier.[219] A trial of this drug is preferred when retained alertness is a goal of therapy.

Octreotide, a somatostatin analog, inhibits gastric, pancreatic, and intestinal secretions and reduces gut motility.[220] Small randomized trials demonstrate its efficacy in relieving the symptoms of malignant bowel obstruction.[221-223] The usual starting dose is 100 mcg twice daily, which may be followed by rapid dose titration.[224] Side effects rarely are a problem, although cost may be a significant issue.

Nonpharmacologic Analgesic Approaches

Although the evidence in support of most nonpharmacologic approaches to pain control is limited, these strategies may be valuable in selected patients.[225] They comprise a diverse group of noninvasive and invasive therapies (**Table 21**). Most are considered adjunctive to a systemic, opioid-based drug regimen.

Interventional Approaches

Interventional approaches comprise a large and varied group of injections, neural blockade approaches, and implant therapies.[84,226] The

Table 21. Pain Treatment Categories for Cancer Populations

Category	Type of Treatment
Pharmacological	Opioid analgesics
	Nonopioid analgesics
	Nontraditional analgesics ("adjuvant analgesics")
Interventional	Injection therapies
	Neural blockade
	Implant therapy
Rehabilitative	Physical modalities such as ultrasound
	Therapeutic exercise
	Occupational therapy
	Hydrotherapy
	Therapy for specific disorders such as lymphedema
Psychological	Psycho-educational interventions
	Cognitive-behavioral therapy
	Relaxation therapy, guided imagery, other types of stress management
	Other forms of psychotherapy
Neurostimulation	Transcutaneous
	Transcranial
	Implanted
Complementary/ Alternative or Integrative	Acupuncture
	Massage
	Physical/movement
	Others

From Treatment of cancer pain, by RK Portenoy, 2011, Lancet, 377(9784), 2236-2247. © 2011 by Elsevier. Reprinted with permission.

simplest are muscle trigger point and joint injections, and local anesthetic infiltration of painful scars.

Neural blockade can be accomplished with local anesthetic (delivered as a bolus or as a perineural infusion) or any of a number of neurolytic approaches (including chemical neurolysis with alcohol or phenol, or mechanical neurolysis using heat or cold).[35] In the past neurolysis was considered for patients with focal or regional pain in the setting of advanced illness and short life expectancy. The advent of nondestructive approaches, such as neuraxial analgesia, has largely supplanted this therapy. At present, only celiac plexus block is commonly performed in medically ill populations. This block can effectively address pain from injury to rostral retroperitoneal structures, such as that caused by pancreatic cancer, and may produce fewer side effects than medications.[227] It may be accomplished using any of a variety of percutaneous needle techniques or via an endoscopic ultrasound-guided approach. Referral to an appropriately trained interventional pain specialist, interventional radiologist, or gastroenterologist[228] usually is necessary.

Placement of an epidural catheter for local anesthetic infusion can be very effective.[84,229] The approach can use low concentrations of anesthetic combined with an opioid and other drugs (known as *neuraxial analgesia*) or aim for anesthesia transiently.[84] An epidural catheter can be percutaneous or tunneled and connected to a port. Placement of a catheter for transient block can be useful in the setting of very severe, opioid-refractory pain. Depending on patient response and other factors, the catheter can be pulled after use, kept in place for a period of time, or used for a trial of neuraxial analgesia later implemented using an implanted intrathecal infusion pump.[230]

In addition to an implanted pump for neuraxial analgesia, implanted neurostimulation therapies are rarely considered for use in patients with opioid-refractory pain.[231] The most common of these therapies, dorsal column stimulation, may be used to treat focal or regional neuropathic pain below the neck.

Other Approaches

Numerous other strategies can be categorized as psychological, rehabilitative, or integrative. Among the most accepted are the mind-body approaches, which are categorized as both psychological and integrative interventions. These treatments should be considered mainstream and are highly useful to address pain and anxiety, enhance coping, and increase self-efficacy.[232] Included among these therapies are interventions that might be encouraged by front-line clinicians, such as relaxation training and guided imagery, and interventions that typically require referral to a trained therapist, such as hypnosis and biofeedback. Relaxation therapy trains patients in a relaxation response induced by repetitive focus on a word, sound, phrase, or body sensation; guided imagery trains patients to recall specific sights, smells, sounds, tastes, or somatic sensations to engender a positive cognitive and emotional state. The strategies can lessen pain[233,234] and confirm the importance of cognitions and emotions as mediators of symptom distress.

Creative art therapies provide another avenue to realize these benefits. These therapies include music,[235] art, and dance[236] and are usually implemented by trained practitioners who become members of the treatment team. These therapies can provide another means to reduce pain while improving coping and adaptation.

Physical modalities are categorized under rehabilitative strategies. Physical modalities comprise the clinical use of heat or cold, electricity, vibration, or ultrasound. They range from the use of ice packs or heating pads to transcutaneous electrical nerve stimulation to deep muscle ultrasound.[237]

Focal musculoskeletal pain is the usual target for these treatments.

Integrative or integrated medicine incorporating complementary or alternative medicine therapies comprise a diverse group of strategies that vary in supporting evidence, familiarity, and use. As noted, the mind-body therapies are mainstream and supported by substantial evidence. Other commonly used approaches in medically ill patients include acupuncture and therapeutic massage and therapies that incorporate physical movement such as tai chi.[238,239] Energy approaches (as defined by the National Institutes of Health National Center for Complementary and Alternative Medicine) such as therapeutic touch are also frequently tried despite minimal evidence of efficacy. Trials of biological substances, often suggested from the perspective of a different system such as Traditional Chinese Medicine, usually are discouraged because of concerns about unanticipated toxicity in the setting of medical illness and the potential for drug-drug interactions. Regardless of the existence of scientific evidence, the use of these approaches is widespread in the United States and clinicians should carefully ask patients about their use.

Management of Procedure-Related Pain

Pain associated with diagnostic and therapeutic procedures may contribute greatly to patient suffering and should be controlled. Specific methods to relieve procedure-related pain are available and should be tailored to the procedure itself.[240] Patient education and sensory preparation, amnestic agents, and analgesic interventions are combined for the best result.[241] It is especially important to control procedure-related pain in children[242] (see *UNIPAC 8*).

Conscious sedation is useful for painful invasive procedures, especially in children. Policies and credentialing are regulated by each healthcare institution. Procedural pain is brief and acute, with little or no time for gradual titration. Become familiar with the administration of opioids and benzodiazepines before attempting to use them to manage procedural pain.[243] Ensure adequate monitoring by skilled personnel other than the person performing the procedure. A healthcare professional skilled in airway management should be present when opioids or sedatives are used for conscious sedation.

Management of Acute Pain Crises

Episodes of acute pain that occur superimposed on a background of otherwise well-managed chronic pain may represent a flare of an underlying painful condition or a new complication and may require urgent intervention. When pain is very severe it should be considered an urgent situation that often requires admission to a hospital bed.

Specific strategies may be considered to address very severe pain. The first approach usually involves rapid opioid titration, either using repeated boluses or a loading infusion approach. Both approaches are best accomplished using a short-acting drug such as morphine, and careful monitoring is required.

Other pharmacologic approaches may be considered. Administration of a corticosteroid at a high dose, such as dexamethasone, 25 mg to 100 mg IV, may be considered for emerging, very severe pain of almost any type. This large loading bolus is followed by a rapid taper as other means of pain control are implemented.

Other nonopioid analgesic drugs can be administered by IV bolus, including acetaminophen and the NSAIDs, ibuprofen or ketorolac. Repeated IV lidocaine boluses also may be considered for neuropathic pain starting at

0.5 mg/kg over 30 minutes. The dose can be doubled and then doubled again at intervals of several hours. Severe neuropathic pain also might be addressed through loading boluses of anticonvulsant drugs[244] with potential analgesic effects, such as valproic acid.

IV ketamine infusion also has gained acceptance as an approach to address emerging severe pain.[245] In a monitoring setting, treatment can begin with a small loading bolus and then infused at a low subanesthethic dose, which is again increased every few hours as needed. If available, interventional therapies such as placement of an epidural or intrathecal catheter for infusion of a local anesthetic and opioid represent additional options to address uncontrolled severe pain.[246]

Finally, when life expectancy is short, severe pain that cannot quickly be controlled in some other way may be the rationale for a discussion about the role of palliative sedation. Recognizing the indications for this therapy, understanding and communicating its medical and ethical basis, and implementing it appropriately are among those skills that specialists in palliative care can bring to a situation that may be generating high distress for patients, families, and the staff members providing care. [247] (See *UNIPAC 6* and the American Academy of Hospice and Palliative Medicine position statement on palliative sedation, available at www.aahpm.org/positions/default/sedation.html.[248])

CLINICAL SITUATION

Joan

Joan is a 66-year-old female with hepatocellular carcinoma at home with hospice. She is currently on morphine extended release 60 mg every 12 hours with morphine elixir 20 mg every 3 hours as needed for pain. She describes her pain as mostly right upper quadrant pain that is constant and increases when she takes a deep breath. It is dull in nature, but with occasional sharp shooting episodes during the day. She is able to ambulate with assistance at home, eat a small amount, and interact with her family. The nurse calls you and reports that Joan is complaining of more right upper quadrant pain that is not relieved with breakthrough medication. She has doubled her breakthrough morphine with little pain relief and resultant somnolence. She asks if there is anything else we can offer for pain?

Question One

What adjuvant pain medications would you consider for Joan? (Choose all that apply.)

A. Acetaminophen, 650 mg every 4 hours as needed for pain

B. Dexamethasone, 4 mg PO twice a day

C. Pamidronate, 90 mg IV

D. Gabapentin, 300 mg PO three times a day

Correct Response and Analysis

B and D are correct answers. Dexamethasone would likely be the best initial choice for liver capsule pain. It may also help associated symptoms such as nausea, anorexia, and depression in patients with advanced disease. Gabapentin is an anticonvulsant medication that is a helpful adjuvant for neuropathic pain. It may take several weeks, however, to titrate up to an effective dose.

A is incorrect because acetaminophen would not likely help liver capsule or neuropathic pain and should be avoided in a patient with liver abnormalities.

C is incorrect because pamidronate is a bisphosphonate that is used primarily for bone pain.

The Case Continues

Joan starts taking scheduled dexamethasone with good results. She has more energy, her appetite increases, and her pain improves for a week. The nurse calls you to report that Joan is sleeping more, eating less, becoming more jaundiced, and is now essentially bedbound. She is grimacing and moving around uncomfortably in bed. The nurse is concerned about the patient not being able to take her extended-release morphine.

Question Two

What would you recommend to the hospice nurse? (Choose all that apply.)

A. Start an SC morphine PCA at 2 mg/hour with 1 mg every 10 minutes as needed.

B. Crush the morpine extended release and give it to the patient in applesauce or pudding.

C. Start a fentanyl patch, 50 mg/hour and continue morphine concentrate for breakthrough.

D. Stop morphine ER and only give morphine concentrate as needed.

Correct Response and Analysis

A and C are correct responses. When patients can no longer take medication by mouth, an alternative route is usually necessary. Options may include an SC PCA with the equivalent dose of continuous IV morphine in the place of morphine extended release. A fentanyl patch may be another valuable alternative, but it has a slow onset of action for this urgent situation.

B is incorrect, because time-release formulations of medications such as morphine ER should not be crushed.

D is incorrect because Joan benefitted from a long-acting opioid for chronic pain, and substituting another long-acting medication via a different route is preferable to just as-needed immediate-release medication. Using scheduled morphine immediate release as a bridge to the transdermal fentanyl might also be effective.

The Case Continues

Joan is started on an SC PCA, and her pain is well-controlled. She is resting comfortably and occasionally wakes up and says a few words or takes a sip of water, then goes back to sleep. Joan's family is worried that she is oversedated. They express concern that the morphine is hastening her death and feel uncomfortable with the "morphine drip."

Question Three

What should be your next response? (Choose all that apply.)

A. Order naloxone and instruct the nurse to push at the bedside.

B. Listen to the family's concerns and explore their underlying fears with the pain medication.

C. Talk to the family about what to expect at the end of life, and explain that for a patient on a stable dose of opioid the risk of oversedation is minimal and that the team is not hastening her death.

D. Rotate her opioid to diladuid, because their main concern is with morphine.

Correct Response and Analysis

Patients with a terminal illness often become less responsive at the end of life. This is a common concern of families at this stage. B and C are the correct answers, because many families do have preconceived ideas about morphine and hastening death. The best approach is to listen to their concerns and explore the reasons behind them. Families need education about what to expect at the end of life, and the role of morphine for comfort.

A and D are incorrect. Naloxone is unnecessary at the end of life and should be used only in rare emergencies where overdose is suspected. Rotation to another opioid does not get to the heart of the issue, which is family understanding and reassurance. A time-limited trial of a lower infusion rate with close observation for signs of distress might also be part of the negotiated plan.

The Case Concludes

The physician and nurse make a home visit and talk to the family about what to expect at the end of life and the role of morphine in the SC route. The family has a better understanding, and they agree to watch closely how a 2 mg/hour morphine infusion rate works. Joan does become more alert but needs more PCA doses for relief, so the family is convinced the medication is necessary. The family spends quality time with her during her last few days at home, and the infusion rate is adjusted as required. Joan dies comfortably while surrounded by family and friends.

Special Populations

Children, frail elderly people, patients with addiction disorders, and marginalized people present special pain management challenges that often result in gross undertreatment. Careful assessments and effective medication dosages are particularly important for these populations.

Assessing Pain in Children

When assessing pain in children, careful attention should be paid to the following issues:
- the child's developmental stage and its effect on the meanings of pain
- the child's developmental stage and its effect on the understanding of the child's prognosis
- the child-parent relationship
- the common occurrence of regression, such as an increased dependence during profound illness.

The high-dose chemotherapy agents used to treat cancer in children often result in treatment-related conditions such as neuropathies, mouth ulcers, and joint pain that may cause more pain than the disease itself, particularly in the case of leukemia.[249] When caring for children, adequately assessing and managing treatment-related sources of pain often is as important as adequately controlling cancer-related pain[250] (see *UNIPAC 8*).

Start with the recommended dosage and rapidly titrate to effect; this often results in a final dosage several times higher than the starting dosage. (For recommended initial opioid dosages for children and more information on pediatric pain management see Table 10 in *UNIPAC 8*.)

Assessing Pain in Elderly Patients

Frail elderly patients often have functional limitations, cognitive deficits, and other comorbidities that require multiple medications. Moderate or higher pain has been shown to be independently associated with frailty.[251] Many clinicians are hesitant to prescribe opioids for this population because they fear precipitating side effects such as delirium, sedation, constipation, and falls. Older patients are generally more susceptible to adverse drug reactions; however, analgesic medications, including opioids, can be used successfully with this population.[252] It is particularly helpful to counsel this population and their family members about the safety and potential side effects of opioids in older patients. Physicians should reassure patients and family members that these side effects are not universal and can be avoided or treated if necessary.[253]

Many drugs and their active or toxic metabolites are cleared by the kidneys. Because reduced renal clearance is common with aging and is a sequelae of many advanced illnesses, clinicians must pay particular attention to renal function.

In frail, older patients, drugs should be started at very low dosages (eg, half the standard adult dosage), such as 2.5 mg of oxycodone. Frequent monitoring should allow careful dose titration if pain is not under control. Side effects should be anticipated and managed preventively when appropriate. Drugs with lesser effects on the CNS, such as nonopioid analgesics or topical agents, should be considered for coanalgesic therapy. Nonpharmacologic strategies also should be used when possible. The addition of these agents and strategies may reduce the overall amount of opioid needed to control a patient's pain.[254]

Patients with Advanced Dementia

Assessing pain can be challenging with patients who have advanced dementia. These patients may have difficulty communicating when experiencing pain. It should be assumed that these patients experience pain, although their ability to process and respond to it often is altered. Instead, they may respond to a noxious stimulus by exhibiting a sudden change in behavior such as physical aggressiveness or social withdrawal.[255,256]

Some patients with advanced dementia can self-report, and it is important to always ask the patient if she or he is feeling pain. Caregivers and family members who know the patient well also can be queried. In nonverbal patients, behavioral indicators such as facial expressions, body movements, vocalizations, and changes in interpersonal interactions or activity patterns may serve as essential data to assess pain[255] (see *UNIPAC 9*).

Several validated assessment tools are available for use with patients who have advanced dementia. The Assessment of Discomfort in Dementia protocol,[257] Discomfort in Dementia of the Alzheimer's Type,[258] and Pain Assessment in Advanced Dementia scale[259] are several examples.

Patients from Diverse Cultures

Analgesic treatment disparities are gaining more attention.[26] Studies of opioid treatment disparities for African Americans remained consistent across pain types, settings, study quality, and data collection periods.[260] The size of the difference was sufficiently large enough to raise not only normative but also quality and safety concerns.[260]

When assessing pain among patients from diverse cultures, careful attention should be paid to the following issues:

- cultural differences in the meanings of pain[261,262]
- cultural differences in religious practices[263]
- cultural expectations regarding reactions to pain, such as stoicism or emotional expression[264,265]
- communication difficulties with non–English-speaking patients.

Patients with Past or Current Substance Use Disorders

A universal precautions approach routinely incorporates the assessment and management of risk associated with drug abuse, addiction, diversion, and overdose when prescribing controlled prescription drugs.[129] Patients with a current or past history of substance abuse are at risk for abuse in the present and can present particular challenges. These challenges do not obviate the need to prescribe adequate dosages of opioids and other analgesics when the appropriate clinical setting exists. Physicians frequently are reluctant to prescribe opioids to patients with a history of addiction or with ongoing addiction issues, and these patients may be equally reluctant and fearful.[266] Such concerns can result in gross undertreatment of patients who are experiencing very severe pain. It is easy to confuse drug-seeking behavior with a legitimate request for relief from uncontrolled pain. Careful assessment is required to establish reliable reports of pain and provide reassurance that appropriate opioid dosages are being prescribed (see *UNIPAC 7*).

Treating pain in patients with past or current drug addictions presents special challenges, but treatment is possible.[267-269] A multidisciplinary approach that includes a mental health provider who has experience with treating drug addiction can assist in both assessment and management of drug-related behavior. A detailed substance-use history is essential and this should include information about social context, duration, frequency, specific drug preferences, and desired effect of drug use. It is important to set realistic goals for therapy. Patients should understand that safe and effective prescribing requires cessation of illicit drug use and increased adherence monitoring as prescribed controlled drugs are used. Comorbid psychiatric disorders including personality disorder, depression, and anxiety should be evaluated and addressed.

Physicians should also consider the therapeutic impact of tolerance. Because opioid abusers may be tolerant of medications prescribed and this tolerance cannot be measured, it is recommended to start conservatively but to rapidly titrate the pain medication dosage and reassess frequently. If concerns about adherence or severe pain complicate the effort to manage drug titration, admission to a monitoring setting may be the safest and best course of action.

Nonadherence behaviors or aberrant drug-related behaviors must be monitored for all patients for whom opioid therapy is pre-scribed (**Table 22**). In ambulatory patients, it is commonplace to obtain urine or saliva drug levels periodically during the course of therapy. If a patient has a history of significant drug abuse, this screening should be done when long-term opioid therapy is initiated, and then considered for repeat testing periodically thereafter. Drug screening should be explained to the patient as part of the standard of care. This conversation need not suggest any lack of trust, but rather, should provide the type of documentation nec-essary for physicians to act consistently in the patient's best interest.

In some cases written statements (medication management or a pain treatment agreement) that explain the roles of team members and

Table 22. Behaviors Suggestive of Addiction

Behaviors Less Indicative of Addiction

- Expressed anxiety or desperation over recurrent symptoms
- Hoarded medications
- Taken someone else's pain medication
- Aggressively complained to the doctor for more drugs
- Requested a specific drug or medication
- Used more opioids than the physician recommended
- Drinks more alcohol when in pain
- Expressed worry over changing to a new drug, even if the drug would have fewer side effects
- Taken someone else's prescription opioids
- Raised opioids dose on their own
- Expressed concern to family, saying that pain might lead to use of street drugs
- Expressed concern to doctor, saying that pain might lead to use of street drugs
- Asked for a second opinion about pain medications
- Smoked cigarettes to relieve pain
- Used opioids to treat other symptoms

Behaviors More Indicative of Addiction

- Bought pain medication from a street dealer
- Stole money to obtain drugs
- Tried to get opioids from more than one source
- Performed sex for drugs
- Seen two doctors at once without them knowing
- Stole drugs from others
- Performed sex for money to obtain drugs
- Selling prescription drugs
- Prostituted others for money to obtain drugs
- Prostituted others for drugs
- Prescription forgery

From Pain and aberrant drug-related behaviors in medically ill patients with and without histories of substance abuse, by SD Passik, KL Kirsh, KB Konaghy, and RK Portenoy, 2006, Clin J Pain, 22, 173-181.[269] © 2006 by Lippincott Williams & Wilkins. Adapted with permission.

the rules and expectations of the patient can be helpful, but they are controversial and there is little evidence that they protect patients or physicians.[270] Patients with aberrant behavior should be seen more frequently and possibly referred to a specialist in addiction medicine.

Patient and Family Education

Patient adherence to a pain management plan improves when healthcare providers take time to listen carefully to the patient's and family's concerns. Concerns about opioid use often are based on common misconceptions (see Clarifying Misconceptions About Opioids). It is important for clinicians to discuss these misconceptions and provide further education about opioids and their treatable side effects. Adherence issues often arise from problems such as swallowing difficulties, concerns about opioid-related constipation, lack of access to expensive medications, and complexity of overall care. Thorough patient and family education is the foundation of effective symptom relief.

Summary

There are reasons to hope for better pain management in the future as research continues and medical evidence accumulates. New pharmacological and nonpharmacological treatments for pain will become available. Standardized measures of clinical outcomes in pain management are being developed that will allow further development of standards of care.

Palliative care specialists are at the forefront of advocacy for the dignity and humane treatment of those with serious life-limiting illnesses and their families. Relieving pain and suffering, regardless of its source, is congruent with our ethic and essential to our task.

References

1. American Pain Society. *Guideline for the Management of Cancer Pain in Adults and Children [Clinical guideline no. 3]*. Glenview, IL: American Pain Society; 2005.

2. Lynn J, Teno JM, Phillips RS, et al. Perceptions by family members of the dying experience of older and seriously ill patients. SUPPORT Investigators. Study to Understand Prognoses and Preferences for Outcomes and Risks of Treatments. *Ann Intern Med.* 1997;126(2):97-106.

3. van den Beuken-van Everdingen MH, de Rijke JM, Kessels AG, Schouten HC, van Kleef M, Patijn J. Prevalence of pain in patients with cancer: a systematic review of the past 40 years. *Ann Oncol.* 2007;18(9):1437-1449.

4. Goudas LC, Bloch R, Gialeli-Goudas M, Lau J, Carr DB. The epidemiology of cancer pain. *Cancer Invest.* 2005;23(2):182-190.

5. World Health Organization. *Cancer Pain Relief with a Guide to Opioid Availability*. 2nd ed. Geneva, Switzerland: World Health Organization; 1996.

6. Benedetti C, Brock C, Cleeland C, et al. NCCN Practice Guidelines for Cancer Pain. *Oncology (Williston Park)*. Nov 2000;14(11A):135-150.

7. Krakowski I, Theobald S, Balp L, et al. Summary version of the Standards, Options and Recommendations for the use of analgesia for the treatment of nociceptive pain in adults with cancer (update 2002). *Br J Cancer.* 2003;89 Suppl 1:S67-72.

8. American Pain Society. *Principles of analgesic use in the treatement of acute pain and cancer pain.* 6th ed. Glenview, IL: American Pain Society; 2008.

9. Jost L, Roila F. Management of cancer pain: ESMO clinical recommendations. *Ann Oncol.* 2008;19 Suppl 2:ii119-121.

10. Cormie PJ, Nairn M, Welsh J. Control of pain in adults with cancer: summary of SIGN guidelines. *BMJ.* 2008;337:a2154.

11. Dy SM, Asch SM, Naeim A, Sanati H, Walling A, Lorenz KA. Evidence-based standards for cancer pain management. *J Clin Oncol.* 2008;26(23):3879-3885.

12. Trescot AM. Review of the role of opioids in cancer pain. *J Natl Compr Canc Netw.* 2010;8(9):1087-1094.

13. Green E, Zwaal C, Beals C, et al. Cancer-related pain management: a report of evidence-based recommendations to guide practice. *Clin J Pain.* 2010;26(6):449-462.

14. Azevedo Sao Leao Ferreira K, Kimura M, Jacobsen Teixeira M. The WHO analgesic ladder for cancer pain control, twenty years of use. How much pain relief does one get from using it? *Support Care Cancer.* 2006;14(11):1086-1093.

15. Oldenmenger WH, Sillevis Smitt PA, van Dooren S, Stoter G, van der Rijt CC. A systematic review on barriers hindering adequate cancer pain management and interventions to reduce them: a critical appraisal. *Eur J Cancer.* 2009;45(8):1370-1380.

16. Deandrea S, Montanari M, Moja L, Apolone G. Prevalence of undertreatment in cancer pain. A review of published literature. *Ann Oncol.* 2008;19(12):1985-1991.

17. Johnson C, Fitzsimmons D, Gilbert J, et al. Development of the European Organisation for Research and Treatment of Cancer quality of life questionnaire module for older people with cancer: The EORTC QLQ-ELD15. *Eur J Cancer.* 2010;46(12):2242-2252.

18. Cassel EJ. The nature of suffering and the goals of medicine. *N Engl J Med.* 1982;306(11):639-645.

19. Cassell EJ. *The Nature of Suffering and the Goals of Medicine.* New York, NY: Oxford University Press; 1991.

20. Wilson KG, Chochinov HM, McPherson CJ, et al. Suffering with advanced cancer. *J Clin Oncol.* 2007;25(13):1691-1697.

21. Ferris FD, Bruera E, Cherny N, et al. Palliative cancer care a decade later: accomplishments, the need, next steps—from the American Society of Clinical Oncology. *J Clin Oncol.* 2009;27(18):3052-3058.

22. Grond S, Zech D, Lynch J, Diefenbach C, Schug SA, Lehmann KA. Validation of World Health Organization guidelines for pain relief in head and neck cancer. A prospective study. *Ann Otol Rhinol Laryngol.* 1993;102(5):342-348.

23. Jadad AR, Browman GP. The WHO analgesic ladder for cancer pain management. Stepping up the quality of its evaluation. *JAMA.* 1995;274(23):1870-1873.

24. Anand A, Carmosino L, Glatt AE. Evaluation of recalcitrant pain in HIV-infected hospitalized patients. *J Acquir Immune Defic Syndr.* 1994;7(1):52-56.

25. National Institutes of Health. *The NIH guide: New Directions in Pain Research I.* Washington, DC: Government Printing Office; 1998.

26. Institute of Medicine. Relieving Pain in America: A Blueprint for Transforming Prevention, Care, Education, and Research. Available at: www.iom.edu/Reports/2011/Relieving-Pain-in-America-A-Blueprint-for-Transforming-Prevention-Care-Education-Research.aspx. Accessed February 3, 2012.

27. Weinstein SM. Nonmalignant pain. In: Walsh DA, Caraceni AT, Fainsinger R, eds. *Palliative Medicine.* 1st ed. Philadelphia, PA: Saunders Elsevier; 2008:931-934.

28. International Association for the Study of Pain. IASP Pain Terminology. In: Merskey H, Bogduk N, eds. *Classification of Chronic Pain.* 2nd ed. Seattle, WA: IASP Press; 1994. www.iasp-pain.org/AM/Template.cfm?Section=General_Resource_Links&Template=/CM/HTMLDisplay.cfm&ContentID=3058#Pain. Accessed January 30, 2012.

29. O'Callaghan JP, Miller DB. Spinal glia and chronic pain. *Metabolism.* 2010;59 Suppl 1:S21-26.

30. Jimenez-Andrade JM, Mantyh WG, Bloom AP, Ferng AS, Geffre CP, Mantyh PW. Bone cancer pain. *Ann N Y Acad Sci.* 2010;1198:173-181.

31. Bennett GJ. Pathophysiology and animal models of cancer-related painful peripheral neuropathy. *Oncologist.* 2010;15 Suppl 2:9-12.

32. Hjermstad MJ, Fainsinger R, Kaasa S. Assessment and classification of cancer pain. *Curr Opin Support Palliat Care.* 2009;3(1):24-30.

33. American Pain Society. APS Glossary of Pain Terminology. APS Pain Society Website. Available at: www.ampainsoc.org/links/pain_glossary.htm. Accessed February 7, 2012.

34. Pereira J. Management of bone pain. In: Portenoy RK, Bruera E, eds. *Topics in Palliative Care.* Vol 3. New York, NY: Oxford University Press; 1998:79-116.

35. Chang VT, Janjan N, Jain S, Chau C. Update in cancer pain syndromes. *J Palliat Med.* 2006;9(6):1414-1434.

36. Elliot K, Foley KM. Neurologic pain syndromes in patients with cancer. In: Portenoy RK, ed. *Pain: Mechanisms and Syndromes, Neurologic Clinics.* Vol 7. Philadelphia, PA: Saunders; 1989:333-360.

37. Portenoy RK. Treatment of cancer pain. *Lancet.* 2011;377(9784):2236-2247.

38. Caraceni A, Portenoy RK. An international survey of cancer pain characteristics and syndromes. IASP Task Force on Cancer Pain. International Association for the Study of Pain. *Pain.* 1999;82(3):263-274.

39. Hicks CL, von Baeyer CL, Spafford PA, van Korlaar I, Goodenough B. The Faces Pain Scale-Revised: toward a common metric in pediatric pain measurement. *Pain.* 2001;93(2):173-183.

40. Hockenberry MJ. *Wong's Essentials of Pediatric Nursing.* 7th ed. St. Louis, MO: Mosby; 2005.

41. Jones KR, Vojir CP, Hutt E, Fink R. Determining mild, moderate, and severe pain equivalency across pain-intensity tools in nursing home residents. *J Rehabil Res Dev.* 2007;44(2):305-314.

42. Holen JC, Hjermstad MJ, Loge JH, et al. Pain assessment tools: is the content appropriate for use in palliative care? *J Pain Symptom Manage.* 2006;32(6):567-580.

43. Melzack R. The McGill Pain Questionnaire: major properties and scoring methods. *Pain.* 1975;1(3):277-299.

44. Gelinas C, Fillion L, Puntillo KA, Viens C, Fortier M. Validation of the critical-care pain observation tool in adult patients. *Am J Crit Care.* 2006;15(4):420-427.

45. Voepel-Lewis T, Zanotti J, Dammeyer JA, Merkel S. Reliability and validity of the face, legs, activity, cry, consolability behavioral tool in assessing acute pain in critically ill patients. *Am J Crit Care.* 2010;19(1):55-61; quiz 62.

46. Puntillo K, Pasero C, Li D, et al. Evaluation of pain in ICU patients. *Chest.* 2009;135(4):1069-1074.

47. Weinstein SM. Physical examination of the patient in pain. In: Ashburn M, ed. *Management of pain.* New York: Churchill Livingston; 1998:17-25.

48. Reddy SK, Weinstein SM. Medical decision-making in a patient with a history of cancer and chronic non-malignant pain. *Clin J Pain.* 1995;11(3):242-246.

49. Piovesan EJ. Diagnostic headache criteria and instruments. In: Herndon RM, ed. *Handbook of Neurologic Rating Scales.* 2nd ed. New York: Demos; 2006:297-345.

50. Morley-Forster P. Prevalence of neuropathic pain and need for treatment. *Pain Research & Management*. 2006 2006;11(Suppl. A):5A-10A.

51. Dworkin RH, Backonja M, Rowbotham MC, et al. Advances in neuropathic pain: diagnosis, mechanisms, and treatment recommendations. *Arch Neurol*. 2003;60(11):1524-1534.

52. Falkmer U, Jarhult J, Wersall P, Cavallin-Stahl E. A systematic overview of radiation therapy effects in skeletal metastases. *Acta Oncol*. 2003;42(5-6):620-633.

53. Tanvetyanon T, Soares HP, Djulbegovic B, Jacobsen PB, Bepler G. A systematic review of quality of life associated with standard chemotherapy regimens for advanced non-small cell lung cancer. *J Thorac Oncol*. 2007;2(12):1091-1097.

54. Cherny NI, Baselga J, de Conno F, Radbruch L. Formulary availability and regulatory barriers to accessibility of opioids for cancer pain in Europe: a report from the ESMO/EAPC Opioid Policy Initiative. *Ann Oncol*. 2010;21(3):615-626.

55. Dworkin RH, O'Connor AB, Backonja M, et al. Pharmacologic management of neuropathic pain: evidence-based recommendations. *Pain*. 2007;132(3):237-251.

56. Lotsch J, Rohrbacher M, Schmidt H, Doehring A, Brockmoller J, Geisslinger G. Can extremely low or high morphine formation from codeine be predicted prior to therapy initiation? *Pain*. 2009;144(1-2):119-124.

57. Klepstad P, Dale O, Kaasa S, et al. Influences on serum concentrations of morphine, M6G and M3G during routine clinical drug monitoring: a prospective survey in 300 adult cancer patients. *Acta Anaesthesiol Scand*. 2003;47(6):725-731.

58. Knotkova H, Fine PG, Portenoy RK. Opioid rotation: the science and the limitations of the equianalgesic dose table. *J Pain Symptom Manage*. 2009;38(3):426-439.

59. Fine PG, Portenoy RK. Establishing "best practices" for opioid rotation: conclusions of an expert panel. *J Pain Symptom Manage*. 2009;38(3):418-425.

60. Maltoni M, Scarpi E, Modonesi C, et al. A validation study of the WHO analgesic ladder: a two-step vs three-step strategy. *Support Care Cancer*. 2005;13(11):888-894.

61. Schneider JP, Matthews M, Jamison RN. Abuse-deterrent and tamper-resistant opioid formulations: what is their role in addressing prescription opioid abuse? *CNS Drugs*. 2010;24(10):805-810.

62. Mercadante S, Radbruch L, Caraceni A, et al. Episodic (breakthrough) pain: consensus conference of an expert working group of the European Association for Palliative Care. *Cancer*. 2002;94(3):832-839.

63. Fine PG, Davies A, Fishman S. *The Diagnosis and Treatment of Breakthrough Pain*. New York, NY: Oxford University Press; 2008.

64. Zeppetella G. Impact and management of breakthrough pain in cancer. *Curr Opin Support Palliat Care*. 2009;3(1):1-6.

65. Aronoff GM, Brennan MJ, Pritchard DD, Ginsberg B. Evidence-based oral transmucosal fentanyl citrate (OTFC) dosing guidelines. *Pain Med*. 2005;6(4):305-314.

66. Coluzzi PH, Schwartzberg L, Conroy JD, et al. Breakthrough cancer pain: a randomized trial comparing oral transmucosal fentanyl citrate (OTFC) and morphine sulfate immediate release (MSIR). *Pain*. 2001;91(1-2):123-130.

67. Mercadante S. Pharmacotherapy for breakthrough cancer pain. *Drugs*. 2012;72(2):181-190.

68. Mercadante S, Ferrera P, Adile C, Casuccio A. Fentanyl buccal tablets for breakthrough pain in highly tolerant cancer patients: preliminary data on the proportionality between breakthrough pain dose and background dose. *J Pain Symptom Manage*. 2011;42(3):464-469.

69. Tassinari D, Sartori S, Tamburini E, et al. Transdermal fentanyl as a front-line approach to moderate-severe pain: a meta-analysis of randomized clinical trials. *J Palliat Care*. 2009;25(3):172-180.

70. Staats PS, Markowitz J, Schein J. Incidence of constipation associated with long-acting opioid therapy: a comparative study. *South Med J*. 2004;97(2):129-134.

71. Gordon DB, Stevenson KK, Griffie J, Muchka S, Rapp C, Ford-Roberts K. Opioid equianalgesic calculations. *J Palliat Med*. 1999;2(2):209-218.

72. Duragesic (fentanyl transdermal system) [package insert].2003; Available at: www.fda.gov/Safety/MedWatch/SafetyInformation/SafetyRelatedDrugLabelingChanges/ucm113224.htm. Accessed February 7, 2012.

73. Skaer TL. Transdermal opioids for cancer pain. *Health Qual Life Outcomes*. 2006;4:24.

74. Hanks GW, Conno F, Cherny N, et al. Morphine and alternative opioids in cancer pain: the EAPC recommendations. *Br J Cancer*. 2001;84(5):587-593.

75. Campiglia L, Cappellini I, Consales G, et al. Premedication with sublingual morphine sulphate in abdominal surgery. *Clin Drug Investig*. 2009;29 Suppl 1:25-30.

76. Kokki H, Rasanen I, Lasalmi M, et al. Comparison of oxycodone pharmacokinetics after buccal and sublingual administration in children. *Clin Pharmacokinet*. 2006;45(7):745-754.

77. Wilkinson TJ, Robinson BA, Begg EJ, Duffull SB, Ravenscroft PJ, Schneider JJ. Pharmacokinetics and efficacy of rectal versus oral sustained-release morphine in cancer patients. *Cancer Chemother Pharmacol*. 1992;31(3):251-254.

78. Bruera E, MacEachern T, Ripamonti C, Hanson J. Subcutaneous morphine for dyspnea in cancer patients. *Ann Intern Med*. 1993;119(9):906-907.

79. Dale O, Sheffels P, Kharasch ED. Bioavailabilities of rectal and oral methadone in healthy subjects. *Br J Clin Pharmacol*. 2004;58(2):156-162.

80. Storey P, Trumble M. Rectal doxepin and carbamazepine therapy in patients with cancer. *N Engl J Med*. 1992;327(18):1318-1319.

81. Pikwer A, Akeson J, Lindgren S. Complications associated with peripheral or central routes for central venous cannulation. *Anaesthesia*. 2012;67(1):65-71.

82. Wilcock A, Jacob JK, Charlesworth S, Harris E, Gibbs M, Allsop H. Drugs given by a syringe driver: a prospective multicentre survey of palliative care services in the UK. *Palliat Med*. 2006;20(7):661-664.

83. Grass JA. Patient-controlled analgesia. *Anesth Analg*. 2005;101(5 Suppl):S44-61.

84. Sloan PA. Neuraxial pain relief for intractable cancer pain. *Curr Pain Headache Rep*. 2007;11(4):283-289.

85. Smith TJ, Staats PS, Deer T, et al. Randomized clinical trial of an implantable drug delivery system compared with comprehensive medical management for refractory cancer pain: impact on pain, drug-related toxicity, and survival. *J Clin Oncol*. 2002;20(19):4040-4049.

86. Cohen SP, Dragovich A. Intrathecal analgesia. *Med Clin North Am*. 2007;91(2):251-270.

87. Burton AW, Rajagopal A, Shah HN, et al. Epidural and intrathecal analgesia is effective in treating refractory cancer pain. *Pain Med*. 2004;5(3):239-247.

88. Mercadante S, Agnello A, Armata MG, Pumo S. The inappropriate use of the epidural route in cancer pain. *J Pain Symptom Manage*. 1997;13(4):233-237.

89. Fainsinger RL, Nekolaichuk CL, Lawlor PG, Neumann CM, Hanson J, Vigano A. A multicenter study of the revised Edmonton Staging System for classifying cancer pain in advanced cancer patients. *J Pain Symptom Manage*. 2005;29(3):224-237.

90. Mercadante S, Bruera E. Opioid switching: a systematic and critical review. *Cancer Treat Rev*. 2006;32(4):304-315.

91. Modesto-Lowe V, Brooks D, Petry N. Methadone deaths: risk factors in pain and addicted populations. *J Gen Intern Med*. 2010;25(4):305-309.

92. Bruera E, Sweeney C. Methadone use in cancer patients with pain: a review. *J Palliat Med*. 2002;5(1):127-138.

93. Iribarne C, Dreano Y, Bardou LG, Menez JF, Berthou F. Interaction of methadone with substrates of human hepatic cytochrome P450 3A4. *Toxicology*. 1997;117(1):13-23.

94. Reddy S, Hui D, El Osta B, et al. The effect of oral methadone on the QTc interval in advanced cancer patients: a prospective pilot study. *Journal of palliative medicine*. 2010;13(1):33-38.

95. Demarie D, Marletta G, Imazio M, et al. Cardiovascular-associated disease in an addicted population: an observation study. *J Cardiovasc Med (Hagerstown)*. 2011;12(1):51-54.

96. Keller GA, Ponte ML, Di Girolamo G. Other drugs acting on nervous system associated with QT-interval prolongation. *Curr Drug Saf*. 2010;5(1):105-111.

97. King S, Forbes K, Hanks GW, Ferro CJ, Chambers EJ. A systematic review of the use of opioid medication for those with moderate to severe cancer pain and renal impairment: a European Palliative Care Research Collaborative opioid guidelines project. *Palliat Med*. 2011;25(5):525-552.

98. Bryson J, Tamber A, Seccareccia D, Zimmermann C. Methadone for treatment of cancer pain. *Curr Oncol Rep*. 2006;8(4):282-288.

99. Sandoval JA, Furlan AD, Mailis-Gagnon A. Oral methadone for chronic noncancer pain: a systematic literature review of reasons for administration,

prescription patterns, effectiveness, and side effects. *Clin J Pain.* 2005;21(6):503-512.

100. Bruera E, Palmer JL, Bosnjak S, et al. Methadone versus morphine as a first-line strong opioid for cancer pain: a randomized, double-blind study. *J Clin Oncol.* 2004;22(1):185-192.

101. Mercadante S, Porzio G, Ferrera P, et al. Sustained-release oral morphine versus transdermal fentanyl and oral methadone in cancer pain management. *Eur J Pain.* 2008;12(8):1040-1046.

102. Mathew P, Storey P. Subcutaneous methadone in terminally ill patients: manageable local toxicity. *J Pain Symptom Manage.* 1999;18(1):49-52.

103. Gazelle G, Fine PG. Fast fact and concept #75: methadone for the treatment of pain. End-of-Life/Palliative Education Resource Center. 2006. 2nd: Available at: www.eperc.mcw.edu/fastfact/ff_75.htm. Accessed February 3, 2012.

104. Ayonrinde OT, Bridge DT. The rediscovery of methadone for cancer pain management. *Med J Aust.* 2000;173(10):536-540.

105. Holzer P, Ahmedzai SH, Niederle N, et al. Opioid-induced bowel dysfunction in cancer-related pain: causes, consequences, and a novel approach for its management. *J Opioid Manag.* 2009;5(3):145-151.

106. Mancini I, Bruera E. Constipation in advanced cancer patients. *Support Care Cancer.* 1998;6(4):356-364.

107. Becker G, Galandi D, Blum HE. Peripherally acting opioid antagonists in the treatment of opiate-related constipation: a systematic review. *J Pain Symptom Manage.* 2007;34(5):547-565.

108. Slatkin NE, Lynn R, Su C, Wang W, Israel RJ. Characterization of abdominal pain during methylnaltrexone treatment of opioid-induced constipation in advanced illness: a post hoc analysis of two clinical trials. *J Pain Symptom Manage.* 2011;42(5):754-760.

109. Jansen JP, Lorch D, Langan J, et al. A randomized, placebo-controlled phase 3 trial (Study SB-767905/012) of alvimopan for opioid-induced bowel dysfunction in patients with non-cancer pain. *J Pain.* 2011;12(2):185-193.

110. Hardy J, Daly S, McQuade B, et al. A double-blind, randomised, parallel group, multinational, multicentre study comparing a single dose of ondansetron 24 mg p.o. with placebo and metoclopramide 10 mg t.d.s. p.o. in the treatment of opioid-induced

nausea and emesis in cancer patients. *Support Care Cancer.* 2002;10(3):231-236.

111. Stone P, Minton O. European Palliative Care Research collaborative pain guidelines. Central side-effects management: what is the evidence to support best practice in the management of sedation, cognitive impairment and myoclonus? *Palliat Med.* 2011;25(5):431-441.

112. Swegle JM, Logemann C. Management of common opioid-induced adverse effects. *Am Fam Physician.* 2006;74(8):1347-1354.

113. Schneider LS, Dagerman KS, Insel P. Risk of death with atypical antipsychotic drug treatment for dementia: meta-analysis of randomized placebo-controlled trials. *JAMA.* 2005;294(15):1934-1943.

114. Schneider LS, Tariot PN, Dagerman KS, et al. Effectiveness of atypical antipsychotic drugs in patients with Alzheimer's disease. *N Engl J Med.* 2006;355(15):1525-1538.

115. Gill SS, Bronskill SE, Normand SL, et al. Antipsychotic drug use and mortality in older adults with dementia. *Ann Intern Med.* 2007;146(11):775-786.

116. Schneeweiss S, Setoguchi S, Brookhart A, Dormuth C, Wang PS. Risk of death associated with the use of conventional versus atypical antipsychotic drugs among elderly patients. *CMAJ.* 2007;176(5):627-632.

117. Dale O, Moksnes K, Kaasa S. European Palliative Care Research Collaborative pain guidelines: opioid switching to improve analgesia or reduce side effects. A systematic review. *Palliat Med.* 2011;25(5):494-503.

118. Cherny N, Ripamonti C, Pereira J, et al. Strategies to manage the adverse effects of oral morphine: an evidence-based report. *J Clin Oncol.* 2001;19(9):2542-2554.

119. Mercadante S. Pathophysiology and treatment of opioid-related myoclonus in cancer patients. *Pain.* 1998;74(1):5-9.

120. Rhodin A, Stridsberg M, Gordh T. Opioid endocrinopathy: a clinical problem in patients with chronic pain and long-term oral opioid treatment. *Clin J Pain.* 2010;26(5):374-380.

121. Walker JM, Farney RJ, Rhondeau SM, et al. Chronic opioid use is a risk factor for the development of central sleep apnea and ataxic breathing. *J Clin Sleep Med.* 2007;3(5):455-461.

122. Chu LF, Angst MS, Clark D. Opioid-induced hyperalgesia in humans: molecular mechanisms and clinical considerations. *Clin J Pain.* 2008;24(6):479-496.

123. Bannister K, Dickenson AH. Opioid hyperalgesia. *Curr Opin Support Palliat Care.* 2010;4(1):1-5.

124. Paulozzi LJ, Kilbourne EM, Shah NG, et al. A history of being prescribed controlled substances and risk of drug overdose death. *Pain Med.* 2012;13(1):87-95.

125. Katz NP, Adams EH, Benneyan JC, et al. Foundations of opioid risk management. *Clin J Pain.* Feb 2007;23(2):103-118.

126. Portenoy RK. Acute and Chronic Pain. In: Ruiz P, Strain, E., ed. *Lowinson & Ruiz's Substance Abuse: A Comprehensive Textbook.* 5th ed. Philadelphia, PA: Lippincott Williams & Wilkins; 2011.

127. Savage SR, Joranson DE, Covington EC, Schnoll SH, Heit HA, Gilson AM. Definitions related to the medical use of opioids: evolution towards universal agreement. *J Pain Symptom Manage.* Jul 2003;26(1):655-667.

128. Portenoy RK. Pain specialists and addiction medicine specialists unite to address critical issues. Available at: www.ampainsoc.org/library/bulletin/mar99/president.htm. Accessed January 31, 2012.

129. Webster LR, Fine PG. Approaches to improve pain relief while minimizing opioid abuse liability. *J Pain.* 2010;11(7):602-611.

130. Clemens KE, Quednau I, Klaschik E. Is there a higher risk of respiratory depression in opioid-naive palliative care patients during symptomatic therapy of dyspnea with strong opioids? *J Palliat Med.* 2008;11(2):204-216.

131. Morita T, Tsunoda J, Inoue S, Chihara S. Effects of high dose opioids and sedatives on survival in terminally ill cancer patients. *J Pain Symptom Manage.* 2001;21(4):282-289.

132. Portenoy RK, Sibirceva U, Smout R, et al. Opioid use and survival at the end of life: a survey of a hospice population. *J Pain Symptom Manage.* 2006;32(6):532-540.

133. Fohr SA. The double effect of pain medication: separating myth from reality. *J Palliat Med.* 1998;1(4):315-328.

134. Axelsson B, Borup S. Is there an additive analgesic effect of paracetamol at step 3? A double-blind randomized controlled study. *Palliat Med.* 2003;17(8):724-725.

135. Stockler M, Vardy J, Pillai A, Warr D. Acetaminophen (paracetamol) improves pain and well-being in people with advanced cancer already receiving a strong opioid regimen: a randomized, double-blind, placebo-controlled cross-over trial. *J Clin Oncol.* 2004;22(16):3389-3394.

136. Israel FJ, Parker G, Charles M, Reymond L. Lack of benefit from paracetamol (acetaminophen) for palliative cancer patients requiring high-dose strong opioids: a randomized, double-blind, placebo-controlled, crossover trial. *J Pain Symptom Manage.* 2010;39(3):548-554.

137. Cubero DI, del Giglio A. Early switching from morphine to methadone is not improved by acetaminophen in the analgesia of oncologic patients: a prospective, randomized, double-blind, placebo-controlled study. *Support Care Cancer.* 2010;18(2):235-242.

138. US Food and Drug Administration. FDA Drug Safety Communication: Prescription Acetaminophen Products to be Limited to 325 mg Per Dosage Unit; Boxed Warning Will Highlight Potential for Severe Liver Failure. Available at: www.fda.gov/Drugs/DrugSafety/ucm239821.htm. Accessed January 31, 2012.

139. Jatox A, Carr DB, Payne R, et al. *Management of Cancer Pain. Clinical Practice Guideline 9. ACHPR Publication 94-0592.* Rockville, MD: Agency for Health Care Policy and Research, US Department of Health and Human Services, Public Health Survey; 1994.

140. Eisenberg E, Berkey CS, Carr DB, Mosteller F, Chalmers TC. Efficacy and safety of nonsteroidal antiinflammatory drugs for cancer pain: a meta-analysis. *J Clin Oncol.* 1994;12(12):2756-2765.

141. McNicol E, Strassels SA, Goudas L, Lau J, Carr DB. NSAIDS or paracetamol, alone or combined with opioids, for cancer pain. *Cochrane Database Syst Rev.* 2005(1):CD005180.

142. Hinz B, Renner B, Brune K. Drug insight: cyclooxygenase-2 inhibitors—a critical appraisal. *Nat Clin Pract Rheumatol.* 2007;3(10):552-560.

143. Lanza FL, Chan FK, Quigley EM. Guidelines for prevention of NSAID-related ulcer complications. *Am J Gastroenterol.* 2009;104(3):728-738.

144. Scheiman JM. Prevention of NSAID-Induced Ulcers. *Curr Treat Options Gastroenterol.* 2008;11(2):125-134.

145. Lazzaroni M, Porro GB. Management of NSAID-induced gastrointestinal toxicity: focus on proton pump inhibitors. *Drugs.* 2009;69(1):51-69.

146. Farkouh ME, Greenberg BP. An evidence-based review of the cardiovascular risks of nonsteroidal anti-inflammatory drugs. *Am J Cardiol.* 2009;103(9):1227-1237.

147. Lussier D, Portenoy RK. Adjuvant analgesics in pain management. In: Hanks G, Cherny N, Christakis N, Kaasa S, Fallon M, Portenoy RK, ed. *Oxford Textbook of Palliative Medicine.* 4th ed. Oxford: Oxford University Press; 2010:706-733.

148. Mercadante S, Portenoy RK. Opioid poorly-responsive cancer pain. Part 3. Clinical strategies to improve opioid responsiveness. *J Pain Symptom Manage.* 2001;21(4):338-354.

149. Della Cuna GR, Pellegrini A, Piazzi M. Effect of methylprednisolone sodium succinate on quality of life in preterminal cancer patients: a placebo-controlled, multicenter study. The Methylprednisolone Preterminal Cancer Study Group. *Eur J Cancer Clin Oncol.* 1989;25(12):1817-1821.

150. Tannock I, Gospodarowicz M, Meakin W, Panzarella T, Stewart L, Rider W. Treatment of metastatic prostatic cancer with low-dose prednisone: evaluation of pain and quality of life as pragmatic indices of response. *J Clin Oncol.* 1989;7(5):590-597.

151. Mercadante SL, Berchovich M, Casuccio A, Fulfaro F, Mangione S. A prospective randomized study of corticosteroids as adjuvant drugs to opioids in advanced cancer patients. *Am J Hosp Palliat Care.* 2007;24(1):13-19.

152. George R, Jeba J, Ramkumar G, Chacko AG, Leng M, Tharyan P. Interventions for the treatment of metastatic extradural spinal cord compression in adults. *Cochrane Database Syst Rev.* 2008(4):CD006716.

153. Verdu B, Decosterd I, Buclin T, Stiefel F, Berney A. Antidepressants for the treatment of chronic pain. *Drugs.* 2008;68(18):2611-2632.

154. Onghena P, Van Houdenhove B. Antidepressant-induced analgesia in chronic non-malignant pain: a meta-analysis of 39 placebo-controlled studies. *Pain.* 1992;49(2):205-219.

155. Collins SL, Moore RA, McQuayHj, Wiffen P. Antidepressants and anticonvulsants for diabetic neuropathy and postherpetic neuralgia: a quantitative systematic review. *J Pain Symptom Manage.* 2000;20(6):449-458.

156. Saarto T, Wiffen PJ. Antidepressants for neuropathic pain. *Cochrane Database Syst Rev.* 2007;(4):CD005454.

157. Sindrup SH, Gram LF, Skjold T, Froland A, Beck-Nielsen H. Concentration-response relationship in imipramine treatment of diabetic neuropathy symptoms. *Clin Pharmacol Ther.* 1990;47(4):509-515.

158. Max MB, Lynch SA, Muir J, Shoaf SE, Smoller B, Dubner R. Effects of desipramine, amitriptyline, and fluoxetine on pain in diabetic neuropathy. *N Engl J Med.* 1992;326(19):1250-1256.

159. Sindrup SH, Bach FW, Madsen C, Gram LF, Jensen TS. Venlafaxine versus imipramine in painful polyneuropathy: a randomized, controlled trial. *Neurology.* 2003;60(8):1284-1289.

160. Rowbotham MC, Goli V, Kunz NR, Lei D. Venlafaxine extended release in the treatment of painful diabetic neuropathy: a double-blind, placebo-controlled study. *Pain.* 2004;110(3):697-706.

161. Arnold LM, Rosen A, Pritchett YL, et al. A randomized, double-blind, placebo-controlled trial of duloxetine in the treatment of women with fibromyalgia with or without major depressive disorder. *Pain.* 2005;119(1-3):5-15.

162. Wernicke JF, Pritchett YL, D'Souza DN, et al. A randomized controlled trial of duloxetine in diabetic peripheral neuropathic pain. *Neurology.* 2006;67(8):1411-1420.

163. Sindrup SH, Gram LF, Brosen K, Eshoj O, Mogensen EF. The selective serotonin reuptake inhibitor paroxetine is effective in the treatment of diabetic neuropathy symptoms. *Pain.* 1990;42(2):135-144.

164. Sindrup SH, Bjerre U, Dejgaard A, Brosen K, Aaes-Jorgensen T, Gram LF. The selective serotonin reuptake inhibitor citalopram relieves the symptoms of diabetic neuropathy. *Clin Pharmacol Ther.* 1992;52(5):547-552.

165. Semenchuk MR, Sherman S, Davis B. Double-blind, randomized trial of bupropion SR for the treatment of neuropathic pain. *Neurology.* 2001;57(9):1583-1588.

166. Eisenach JC, DuPen S, Dubois M, Miguel R, Allin D. Epidural clonidine analgesia for intractable cancer pain. The Epidural Clonidine Study Group. *Pain.* 1995;61(3):391-399.

167. Malanga GA, Gwynn MW, Smith R, Miller D. Tizanidine is effective in the treatment of myofascial pain syndrome. *Pain Physician.* 2002;5(4):422-432.

168. Arain SR, Ruehlow RM, Uhrich TD, Ebert TJ. The efficacy of dexmedetomidine versus morphine for postoperative analgesia after major inpatient surgery. *Anesth Analg.* 2004;98(1):153-158.

169. Skrabek RQ, Galimova L, Ethans K, Perry D. Nabilone for the treatment of pain in fibromyalgia. *J Pain.* Feb 2008;9(2):164-173.

170. Svendsen KB, Jensen TS, Bach FW. Does the cannabinoid dronabinol reduce central pain in multiple sclerosis? Randomised double blind placebo controlled crossover trial. *BMJ.* Jul 31 2004;329(7460):253.

171. Rog DJ, Nurmikko TJ, Friede T, Young CA. Randomized, controlled trial of cannabis-based medicine in central pain in multiple sclerosis. *Neurology.* 2005;65(6):812-819.

172. Russo EB, Guy GW, Robson PJ. Cannabis, pain, and sleep: lessons from therapeutic clinical trials of Sativex, a cannabis-based medicine. *Chem Biodivers.* 2007;4(8):1729-1743.

173. Novotna A, Mares J, Ratcliffe S, et al. A randomized, double-blind, placebo-controlled, parallel-group, enriched-design study of nabiximols* (Sativex®), as add-on therapy, in subjects with refractory spasticity caused by multiple sclerosis. *Eur J Neurol.* 2011;18(9):1122-1131.

174. Galer BS, Rowbotham MC, Perander J, Friedman E. Topical lidocaine patch relieves postherpetic neuralgia more effectively than a vehicle topical patch: results of an enriched enrollment study. *Pain.* 1999;80(3):533-538.

175. Rowbotham MC, Davies PS, Fields HL. Topical lidocaine gel relieves postherpetic neuralgia. *Ann Neurol.* 1995;37(2):246-253.

176. Stow PJ, Glynn CJ, Minor B. EMLA cream in the treatment of post-herpetic neuralgia. Efficacy and pharmacokinetic profile. *Pain.* 1989;39(3):301-305.

177. Barbano RL, Herrmann DN, Hart-Gouleau S, Pennella-Vaughan J, Lodewick PA, Dworkin RH. Effectiveness, tolerability, and impact on quality of life of the 5% lidocaine patch in diabetic polyneuropathy. *Arch Neurol.* 2004;61(6):914-918.

178. Gammaitoni AR, Galer BS, Onawola R, Jensen MP, Argoff CE. Lidocaine patch 5% and its positive impact on pain qualities in osteoarthritis:

results of a pilot 2-week, open-label study using the Neuropathic Pain Scale. *Curr Med Res Opin.* 2004;20 Suppl 2:S13-19.

179. Gammaitoni AR, Alvarez NA, Galer BS. Pharmacokinetics and safety of continuously applied lidocaine patches 5%. *Am J Health Syst Pharm.* 2002;59(22):2215-2220.

180. Knotkova H, Pappagallo M, Szallasi A. Capsaicin (TRPV1 Agonist) therapy for pain relief: farewell or revival? *Clin J Pain.* 2008;24(2):142-154.

181. US Food and Drug Administration. FDA approves new drug treatment for long-term pain relief after shingles attacks. Available at: www.fda.gov/NewsEvents/Newsroom/PressAnnouncements/2009/ucm191003.htm. Accessed January 31, 2012.

182. Lin J, Zhang W, Jones A, Doherty M. Efficacy of topical non-steroidal anti-inflammatory drugs in the treatment of osteoarthritis: meta-analysis of randomised controlled trials. *BMJ.* 2004;329(7461):324.

183. Ho KY, Huh BK, White WD, Yeh CC, Miller EJ. Topical amitriptyline versus lidocaine in the treatment of neuropathic pain. *Clin J Pain.* 2008;24(1):51-55.

184. National Comprehensive Cancer Network (NCCN). Clinical Practice Guidelines for Cancer Pain, version 2.2011. Available at: www.nccn.org/professionals/physician_gls/pdf/pain.pdf. Accessed January 31, 2012.

185. Serpell MG. Gabapentin in neuropathic pain syndromes: a randomised, double-blind, placebo-controlled trial. *Pain.* 2002;99(3):557-566.

186. Caraceni A, Zecca E, Bonezzi C, et al. Gabapentin for neuropathic cancer pain: a randomized controlled trial from the Gabapentin Cancer Pain Study Group. *J Clin Oncol.* 2004;22(14):2909-2917.

187. Frampton JE, Foster RH. Pregabalin: in the treatment of postherpetic neuralgia. *Drugs.* 2005;65(1):111-118.

188. Dworkin RH, Corbin AE, Young JP, Jr., et al. Pregabalin for the treatment of postherpetic neuralgia: a randomized, placebo-controlled trial. *Neurology.* 2003;60(8):1274-1283.

189. Rosenstock J, Tuchman M, LaMoreaux L, Sharma U. Pregabalin for the treatment of painful diabetic peripheral neuropathy: a double-blind, placebo-controlled trial. *Pain.* 2004;110(3):628-638.

190. Wiffen PJ, McQuay HJ, Edwards JE, Moore RA. Gabapentin for acute and chronic pain. *Cochrane Database Syst Rev.* 2005(3):CD005452.

191. Vondracek P, Oslejskova H, Kepak T, et al. Efficacy of pregabalin in neuropathic pain in paediatric oncological patients. *Eur J Paediatr Neurol.* 2009;13(4):332-336.

192. Moore RA, Wiffen PJ, Derry S, McQuay HJ. Gabapentin for chronic neuropathic pain and fibromyalgia in adults. *Cochrane Database Syst Rev.* 2011;(3):CD007938.

193. Toth C. Substitution of gabapentin therapy with pregabalin therapy in neuropathic pain due to peripheral neuropathy. *Pain Med.* 2010;11(3):456-465.

194. Eisenberg E, River Y, Shifrin A, Krivoy N. Antiepileptic drugs in the treatment of neuropathic pain. *Drugs.* 2007;67(9):1265-1289.

195. Wiffen PJ, McQuay HJ, Moore RA. Carbamazepine for acute and chronic pain. *Cochrane Database Syst Rev.* 2005;(3):CD005451.

196. Wiffen PJ, Rees J. Lamotrigine for acute and chronic pain. *Cochrane Database Syst Rev.* 2007;(2):CD006044.

197. Nasreddine W, Beydoun A. Oxcarbazepine in neuropathic pain. *Expert Opin Investig Drugs.* 2007;16(10):1615-1625.

198. Bendaly EA, Jordan CA, Staehler SS, Rushing DA. Topiramate in the treatment of neuropathic pain in patients with cancer. *Support Cancer Ther.* 2007;4(4):241-246.

199. Wymer JP, Simpson J, Sen D, Bongardt S. Efficacy and safety of lacosamide in diabetic neuropathic pain: an 18-week double-blind placebo-controlled trial of fixed-dose regimens. *Clin J Pain.* 2009;25(5):376-385.

200. Hugel H, Ellershaw JE, Dickman A. Clonazepam as an adjuvant analgesic in patients with cancer-related neuropathic pain. *J Pain Symptom Manage.* 2003;26(6):1073-1074.

201. Tremont-Lukats IW, Challapalli V, McNicol ED, Lau J, Carr DB. Systemic administration of local anesthetics to relieve neuropathic pain: a systematic review and meta-analysis. *Anesth Analg.* 2005;101(6):1738-1749.

202. Challapalli V, Tremont-Lukats IW, McNicol ED, Lau J, Carr DB. Systemic administration of local anesthetic agents to relieve neuropathic pain. *Cochrane Database Syst Rev.* 2005;(4):CD003345.

203. Dworkin RH, O'Connor AB, Audette J, et al. Recommendations for the pharmacological management of neuropathic pain: an overview and literature update. *Mayo Clin Proc.* 2010;85(3 Suppl):S3-14.

204. Bell R, Eccleston C, Kalso E. Ketamine as an adjuvant to opioids for cancer pain. *Cochrane Database Syst Rev.* 2003;(1):CD003351.

205. Ben-Ari A, Lewis MC, Davidson E. Chronic administration of ketamine for analgesia. *J Pain Palliat Care Pharmacother.* 2007;21(1):7-14.

206. Chizh BA, Headley PM. NMDA antagonists and neuropathic pain—multiple drug targets and multiple uses. *Curr Pharm Des.* 2005;11(23):2977-2994.

207. Yomiya K, Matsuo N, Tomiyasu S, et al. Baclofen as an adjuvant analgesic for cancer pain. *Am J Hosp Palliat Care.* 2009;26(2):112-118.

208. Costa L, Major PP. Effect of bisphosphonates on pain and quality of life in patients with bone metastases. *Nat Clin Pract Oncol.* 2009;6(3):163-174.

209. Miksad RA, Lai KC, Dodson TB, et al. Quality of life implications of bisphosphonate-associated osteonecrosis of the jaw. *Oncologist.* 2011;16(1):121-132.

210. Park-Wyllie LY, Mamdani MM, Juurlink DN, et al. Bisphosphonate use and the risk of subtrochanteric or femoral shaft fractures in older women. *JAMA.* 2011;305(8):783-789.

211. Van Poznak CH, Temin S, Yee GC, et al. American Society of Clinical Oncology executive summary of the clinical practice guideline update on the role of bone-modifying agents in metastatic breast cancer. *J Clin Oncol.* 2011;29(9):1221-1227.

212. Martinez-Zapata MJ, Roque M, Alonso-Coello P, Catala E. Calcitonin for metastatic bone pain. *Cochrane Database Syst Rev.* 2006;3:CD003223.

213. Christensen MH, Petersen LJ. Radionuclide treatment of painful bone metastases in patients with breast cancer: A systematic review. *Cancer Treat Res.* 2012;38(2):164-171.

214. Roque IFM, Martinez-Zapata MJ, Scott-Brown M, Alonso-Coello P. Radioisotopes for metastatic bone pain. *Cochrane Database Syst Rev.* 2011;(7):CD003347.

215. Frech EJ, Adler DG. Endoscopic therapy for malignant bowel obstruction. *J Support Oncol.* 2007;5(7):303-310, 319.

216. Kucukmetin A, Naik R, Galaal K, Bryant A, Dickinson HO. Palliative surgery versus medical management for bowel obstruction in ovarian cancer. *Cochrane Database Syst Rev.* 2010;(7):CD007792.

217. Laval G, Girardier J, Lassauniere JM, Leduc B, Haond C, Schaerer R. The use of steroids in the management of inoperable intestinal obstruction in terminal cancer patients: do they remove the obstruction? *Palliat Med.* 2000;14(1):3-10.

218. Feuer DJ, Broadley KE. Systematic review and meta-analysis of corticosteroids for the resolution of malignant bowel obstruction in advanced gynaecological and gastrointestinal cancers. Systematic Review Steering Committee. *Ann Oncol.* 1999;10(9):1035-1041.

219. Davis MP, Furste A. Glycopyrrolate: a useful drug in the palliation of mechanical bowel obstruction. *J Pain Symptom Manage.* 1999;18(3):153-154.

220. Dean A. The palliative effects of octreotide in cancer patients. *Chemotherapy.* 2001;47 Suppl 2:54-61.

221. Ripamonti C, Mercadante S, Groff L, Zecca E, De Conno F, Casuccio A. Role of octreotide, scopolamine butylbromide, and hydration in symptom control of patients with inoperable bowel obstruction and nasogastric tubes: a prospective randomized trial. *J Pain Symptom Manage.* 2000;19(1):23-34.

222. Mercadante S, Ripamonti C, Casuccio A, Zecca E, Groff L. Comparison of octreotide and hyoscine butylbromide in controlling gastrointestinal symptoms due to malignant inoperable bowel obstruction. *Support Care Cancer.* 2000;8(3):188-191.

223. Mystakidou K, Tsilika E, Kalaidopoulou O, Chondros K, Georgaki S, Papadimitriou L. Comparison of octreotide administration vs conservative treatment in the management of inoperable bowel obstruction in patients with far advanced cancer: a randomized, double-blind, controlled clinical trial. *Anticancer Res.* 2002;22(2B):1187-1192.

224. Murphy E, Prommer EE, Mihalyo M, Wilcock A. Octreotide. *J Pain Symptom Manage.* 2010;40(1):142-148.

225. Blaes AH, Kreitzer MJ, Torkelson C, Haddad T. Nonpharmacologic complementary therapies in symptom management for breast cancer survivors. *Semin Oncol.* 2011;38(3):394-402.

226. Brogan S, Junkins S. Interventional therapies for the management of cancer pain. *J Support Oncol.* 2010;8(2):52-59.

227. Arcidiacono PG, Calori G, Carrara S, McNicol ED, Testoni PA. Celiac plexus block for pancreatic cancer pain in adults. *Cochrane Database Syst Rev.* 2011(3):CD007519.

228. Kaufman M, Singh G, Das S, et al. Efficacy of endoscopic ultrasound-guided celiac plexus block and celiac plexus neurolysis for managing abdominal pain associated with chronic pancreatitis and pancreatic cancer. *J Clin Gastroenterol.* 2010;44(2):127-134.

229. Ballantyne JC, Carwood CM. Comparative efficacy of epidural, subarachnoid, and intracerebroventricular opioids in patients with pain due to cancer. *Cochrane Database Syst Rev.* 2005;(1):CD005178.

230. Stearns L, Boortz-Marx R, Du Pen S, et al. Intrathecal drug delivery for the management of cancer pain: a multidisciplinary consensus of best clinical practices. *J Support Oncol.* 2005;3(6):399-408.

231. Yakovlev AE, Resch BE, Karasev SA. Treatment of cancer-related chest wall pain using spinal cord stimulation. *Am J Hosp Palliat Care.* 2010;27(8):552-556.

232. Carnes D, Homer KE, Miles CL, et al. Effective delivery styles and content for self-management interventions for chronic musculoskeletal pain: a systematic literature review. *Clin J Pain.* Epub Oct 13 2011.

233. Kwekkeboom KL, Cherwin CH, Lee JW, Wanta B. Mind-body treatments for the pain-fatigue-sleep disturbance symptom cluster in persons with cancer. *J Pain Symptom Manage.* 2010;39(1):126-138.

234. Bardia A, Barton DL, Prokop LJ, Bauer BA, Moynihan TJ. Efficacy of complementary and alternative medicine therapies in relieving cancer pain: a systematic review. *J Clin Oncol.* 2006;24(34):5457-5464.

235. Bradt J, Dileo C, Grocke D, Magill L. Music interventions for improving psychological and physical outcomes in cancer patients. *Cochrane Database Syst Rev.* 2011;(8):CD006911.

236. Bradt J, Goodill SW, Dileo C. Dance/movement therapy for improving psychological and physical outcomes in cancer patients. *Cochrane Database Syst Rev.* 2011;(10):CD007103.

237. Srbely JZ, Dickey JP. Randomized controlled study of the antinociceptive effect of ultrasound on trigger point sensitivity: novel applications in myofascial therapy? *Clin Rehabil.* 2007;21(5):411-417.

238. Ernst E. Massage therapy for cancer palliation and supportive care: a systematic review of randomised clinical trials. *Support Care Cancer.* 2009;17(4):333-337.

239. Wang C, Schmid CH, Rones R, et al. A randomized trial of tai chi for fibromyalgia. *N Engl J Med.* 2010;363(8):743-754.

240. Swarm R, Abernethy AP, Anghelescu DL, et al. Adult cancer pain. *J Natl Compr Canc Netw.* 2010;8(9):1046-1086.

241. Moreno MA, Furtner F, Rivara FP. How parents can help children cope with procedures and pain. *Arch Pediatr Adolesc Med.* 2011;165(9):872.

242. Accardi MC, Milling LS. The effectiveness of hypnosis for reducing procedure-related pain in children and adolescents: a comprehensive methodological review. *J Behav Med.* 2009;32(4):328-339.

243. Guideline for monitoring and management of pediatric patients during and after sedation for diagnostic and therapeutic procedures. *Pediatric Dent.* 2008;30(7 Suppl):143-159.

244. Cheshire WP. Fosphenytoin: an intravenous option for the management of acute trigeminal neuralgia crisis. *J Pain Symptom Manage.* 2001;21(6):506-510.

245. Meals CG, Mullican BD, Shaffer CM, Dangerfield PF, Ramirez RP. Ketamine infusion for sickle cell crisis pain in an adult. *J Pain Symptom Manage.* 2011;42(3):e7-9.

246. McHardy P, McDonnell C, Lorenzo AJ, Salle JL, Campbell FA. Management of priapism in a child with sickle cell anemia; successful outcome using epidural analgesia. *Can J Anaesth.* 2007;54(8):642-645.

247. Levy MH, Back A, Benedetti C, et al. NCCN clinical practice guidelines in oncology: palliative care. *J Natl Compr Canc Netw.* 2009;7(4):436-473.

248. American Academy of Hospice and Palliative Medicine. Statement on Palliative Sedation. Available at: www.aahpm.org/positions/default/sedation.html. Accessed January 30, 2012.

249. Poder U, Ljungman G, von Essen L. Parents' perceptions of their children's cancer-related symptoms during treatment: a prospective, longitudinal study. *J Pain Symptom Manage.* 2010;40(5):661-670.

250. Po C, Benini F, Sainati L, Farina MI, Cesaro S, Agosto C. The management of procedural pain at the Italian Centers of Pediatric Hematology-Oncology: state-of-the-art and future directions. *Support Care Cancer.* Epub Dec 31 2011.

251. Shega JW, Dale W, Andrew M, Paice J, Rockwood K, Weiner DK. Persistent pain and frailty: a case for homeostenosis. *J Am Geriatr Soc.* 2012;60(1):113-117.

252. Schmader KE, Baron R, Haanpaa ML, et al. Treatment considerations for elderly and frail patients with neuropathic pain. *Mayo Clin Proc.* 2010;85(3 Suppl):S26-32.

253. McLachlan AJ, Bath S, Naganathan V, et al. Clinical pharmacology of analgesic medicines in older people: impact of frailty and cognitive impairment. *Br J Clin Pharmacol.* 2011;71(3):351-364.

254. Pharmacological management of persistent pain in older persons. *J Am Geriatr Soc.* 2009;57(8):1331-1346.

255. Herr K, Bjoro K, Decker S. Tools for assessment of pain in nonverbal older adults with dementia: a state-of-the-science review. *J Pain Symptom Manage.* 2006;31(2):170-192.

256. Gibson SJ. What does an increased prevalence of behavioral and psychological symptoms of dementia in individuals with pain mean? *Pain.* 2012;153(2):261-262.

257. Kovach CR, Weissman DE, Griffie J, Matson S, Muchka S. Assessment and treatment of discomfort for people with late-stage dementia. *J Pain Symptom Manage.* 1999;18(6):412-419.

258. Hurley AC, Volicer BJ, Hanrahan PA, Houde S, Volicer L. Assessment of discomfort in advanced Alzheimer patients. *Res Nurs Health.* 1992;15(5):369-377.

259. Warden V, Hurley AC, Volicer L. Development and psychometric evaluation of the Pain Assessment in Advanced Dementia (PAINAD) scale. *J Am Med Dir Assoc.* 2003;4(1):9-15.

260. Meghani SH, Byun E, Gallagher RM. Time to take stock: a meta-analysis and systematic review of analgesic treatment disparities for pain in the United States. *Pain Med.* Epub Jan. 13 2012.

261. Ozkan S, Ozkan M, Armay Z. Cultural meaning of cancer suffering. *J Pediatr Hematol Oncol.* 2011;33 Suppl 2:S102-104.

262. Magnusson JE, Fennell JA. Understanding the role of culture in pain: Maori practitioner perspectives relating to the experience of pain. *N Z Med J.* 2011;124(1328):41-51.

263. Delgado-Guay MO, Hui D, Parsons HA, et al. Spirituality, religiosity, and spiritual pain in advanced cancer patients. *J Pain Symptom Manage*. 2011;41(6):986-994.

264. Chen CH, Tang ST. Meta-analysis of cultural differences in Western and Asian patient-perceived barriers to managing cancer pain. *Palliat Med*. Epub Apr 7 2011.

265. Wein S. Impact of culture on the expression of pain and suffering. *J Pediatr Hematol Oncol*. 2011;33 Suppl 2:S105-107.

266. Gonzales GR, Coyle N. Treatment of cancer pain in a former opioid abuser: fears of the patient and staff and their influence on care. *J Pain Symptom Manage*. 1992;7(4):246-249.

267. Robb V. Working on the edge: palliative care for substance users with AIDS. *J Palliat Care*. 1995;11(2):50-53.

268. Kirsh KL, Passik SD. Palliative care of the terminally ill drug addict. *Cancer Invest*. 2006;24(4):425-431.

269. Passik SD, Kirsh KL, Donaghy KB, Portenoy RK. Pain and aberrant drug-related behaviors in medically ill patients with and without histories of substance abuse. *Clin J Pain*. 2006;22(2):173-181.

270. Payne R, Anderson E, Arnold R, et al. A rose by any other name: pain contracts/agreements. *Am J Bioeth*. 2010;10(11):5-12.

Index

A

A-delta fibers, 5
acetaminophen, 43–44
    characteristics of, 45t
    contraindications, 44
    dosage, 43–44
    hydrocodone with, 29
    pain treatment with, 18, 57
acetic acids, characteristics of, 46t
acetylsalicylic acid, 45t
acupressure, for constipation, 37
acupuncture, for constipation, 37
acute pain crises, management of, 57–58
addiction, 62–64
    behaviors suggestive of, 63t
    definition of, 39
    opioids and, 40–42
alpha-2-adrenergic agonists, 49t, 51
alvimopan, 36
amantadine, 54
amitriptyline, 49t, 50
analgesia
    adjuvant, 47–55
    equianalgesia guidelines, 22t
    multipurpose, 48–52, 49t
    nonpharmacologic, 55–57
analgesic ladder (WHO), 17–19, 19f
anorexia, glucocorticoids for, 48
anticholinergic drugs, 55
anticonvulsants, 52–53
antidepressants
    analgesic action of, 48–51, 49t, 50
    analgesics and, 48
antiemetics, 26, 36
anxiety, pain and, 1t
aspirin, 44, 45t

B

baclofen, 50t
benzodiazepines, 37
beta endorphin, 5
bisacodyl, 35, 36

bisphosphonates, 50t, 54
bone pain
    drug selection, 54
    movement and, 7
    tumor-related, 9t
bowel obstruction, 55
breakthrough doses, 23
breakthrough pain
    drugs for, 22–23
    episodes of, 14
    types of, 23t
Brief Pain Inventory (BPI), 12
buprenorphine, 19, 24–25
bupropion, 49t, 50
butorphanol, 19

C

C-fibers, 5
calcitonin, 54
cancer pain, 1, 17, 55t
cannabinoids, 48, 49t, 51–52
capsaicin, 52
carbamazepine, 49t, 53
catheters, epidural, 56
celecoxib, 44, 46t
chemotherapy, pain-related to, 10t, 61
children, pain management, 61
choline magnesium trisalicylate, 44, 45t
chronic nonmalignant pain, 3t
chronic pain
    incidence of, 3
    pathophysiology, 5–6
chronic pain syndromes, 9t–10t
citalopram, 49t
clodronate, 50t, 54
clonazepam, 37, 50t, 53
clonidine, 49t
codeine
    equianalgesic dose tables, 20t
    pain treatment with, 18
    selection of, 19
cognitive strategies, 37

H

haloperidol, 26, 36, 37
headache, pain of, 3
heart rates, pain and, 14
heating pads, 57
hopelessness, pain and, 1t
hyaluronidase, 26
hydration, SC administration, 26
hydrocodone, 18, 20t, 29
hydromorphone
    dosage, 23
    equianalgesic dose tables, 20t
    immediate-release, 25
    starting dosages, 29
hyperalgesia, opioid-induced, 34, 38–39
hypertension, pain and, 14
hypodermoclysis, 26
hypogonadism, opioid-induced, 38

I

ibandronate, 50t, 54
ibuprofen
    characteristics of, 45t
    pain treatment with, 57
    side effects, 44
ice packs, 57
indomethacin, 46t
intensive care units (ICUs), 12–13
International Association for the Study of Pain, 5
interpersonal problems, 1t
intravenous administration, 25

K

kappa receptors, 5
ketamine, 50t, 52, 53, 58
ketoprofen, 45t
ketorolac, 46t, 57

L

lacosamide, 49t, 50t, 53
lactulose, 35
lamotrigine, 49t, 53
language barriers, 12
laxatives, stepwise regimen, 35t
lidocaine, 49t, 52, 57
lower back pain, 3

M

malaise, glucocorticoids for, 48
McGill Pain Questionnaire (MPQ), 12
meclizine, 36
meclofenamic acid, 46t
mefenamic acid, 46t
memantine, 50t, 54
mental clouding, opioid-related, 37
meperidine, 19, 20t
metaclopramide, 26, 36
methadone
    accumulation of, 21t
    cautions about, 21t
    conversion of, 33t
    drug interactions, 21t
    equianalgesic dose tables, 20t
    half-life, 21t
    IV to oral conversion, 21t
    NMDA receptors blockage by, 32
    oral to IV conversion, 21t
    pain treatment with, 18
    rectal administration, 25
    rotation, 31–32
    sublingual administration, 24–25
N-methyl-D-aspartrate (NMDA) inhibitors, 50t
N-methyl-D-aspartrate (NMDA) receptors, 32
methylnaltrexone, 36
methylphenidate, 37
mexiletine, 49t, 53
milnacipran, 49t, 51
modafinil, 37
morphine
    administration of, 26
    conversion of, 33t
    dosages, 23, 25t, 31, 59
    equianalgesic dose tables, 20t
    immediate-release, 25
    modified-release, 22, 23
    pain treatment with, 18
    pulsed administration, 28
    rectal administration, 25
    selection of, 19
    starting dosages, 29
mu-agonist opioids, 18, 19
mu receptors, 5

musculoskeletal examination, 15*t*

myelosuppression, 54

myoclonus, 34, 37

N

nabilone, 49*t*

nabiximols, 52

nabumetone, 44, 47*t*

naloxone (Narcan), 22*t*

naphthlalkanones, 47*t*

naproxen

    characteristics of, 45*t*

    rectal administration, 25

    side effects, 44, 47

nausea, glucocorticoids for, 48

nausea and vomiting

    movement-related, 36

    opioid-related, 36–37

    post-prandial, 36

neural blockade, 56

neuraxial analgesia, 27

neurological examination, 15*t*

neuropathic pain, 8, 52–54

neurotransmitter release, 5

nociceptive pain, 6, 9*t*

nociceptors, 5

nonadherence behaviors, 63

nonmalignant pain, 3, 3*t*

nonopioid analgesics, 43–47

nonsteroidal anti-inflammatory drugs (NSAIDs), 44–47

    characteristics of, 45*t*–47*t*

    pain treatment with, 18

    side effects, 44

nortriptyline, 50

O

octreotide, 50*t*, 55

olanzepine, 36, 37

omeprazole, 36

ondansetron, 36

opioid analgesics, 19–23

    dose titration, 29–30

    drug selection, 19–22

    guidelines, 31*t*

    hastened death and, 42–43

opioid analgesics *(cont.)*

    misconceptions, 40–43

    overdoses, 37–38

    pain treatment with, 2, 18

    poor responsiveness, 30*t*

    potencies, 27*t*

    regulatory scrutiny, 2

    risk management, 39–40, 41*t*–42*t*

    rotation of, 30–33, 31*t*, 33*t*

    side effects, 33–39

    starting dosages, 29–30

    tolerance and, 42

    withholding of, 42–43

opioid-induced hyperalgesia (OIH), 34, 38–39

opioid receptors, 5

opioid rotation, 19

oral route, 33*t*

oxaprozin, 45*t*

oxcarbazepine, 49*t*, 53

oxicam, 46*t*

oxycodone

    equianalgesic dose tables, 20*t*

    extended-release, 28

    immediate-release, 25

    modified-release, 22

    pain treatment with, 18

    starting dosages, 29

oxymorphone, 18

P

pain

    barriers to treatment of, 1

    definition of, 5

    diagnostic testing, 16*t*

    inappropriate care, 1

    nomenclature, 5–10

    nonphysical, 1–2

    pathophysiology, 5–10

    physical, 1–2

    procedural, 2

    sources of, 3

    undertreatment, 2

pain assessment, 6–8, 11–16

    components of, 11–16

    history in, 14